The Arthritic's Book of
WATER EXERCISE

The Arthritic's Book of
WATER EXERCISE

Judy Jetter and Nancy Kadlec

GRANADA
London Toronto Sydney New York

Granada Publishing Limited
8 Grafton Street, London W1X 3LA

Published in the USA by Holt, Rinehart and Winston 1985
Published in Great Britain by Granada Publishing 1985

Text copyright © Judy Jetter and Nancy Kadlec 1985

Photographs copyright © Michael Hoffman 1985

British Library Cataloguing in Publication Data

Jetter, Judy
  The arthritic's book of water exercise.
  1. Arthritis – Treatment   2. Hydrotherapy
  I. Title   II. Kadlec, Nancy
  616.7'220653   RC933

ISBN 0–246–12684–1

Printed in Great Britain by
Mackays of Chatham Limited

CONTENTS

To our many friends with 'rusty hinges'
for their unwavering support, and to
the Arthritis Foundation for their
thoughtful praise and encouragement.

FOREWORD

by F. Dudley Hart, MD, FRCP
Consulting Physician, Westminster Hospital, and the
Hospital of St John and St Elizabeth, London

I am very happy to write a foreword for this book as the authors have produced a useful and practical work for arthritic patients to help them help themselves. There is no doubt that exercises in water enable the arthritic patient to maintain and extend his or her mobility, increase his or her strength and lessen pain. The realization that more can be done with less discomfort in water acts not only as a great physical stimulus but as a psychological one also, for fighting arthritis can be a depressing and soul-destroying affair which all too often appears to go on and on without respite.

As the authors of this excellent book say, there are well over a hundred conditions affecting muscles, bones and joints which come under the general heading of arthritis or rheumatism, some of which are serious and severe, some only a major nuisance, but all of which are painful. Exercises in water are popular with my patients, most of whom gain considerable benefit from them. The exercises clearly explained here cover all conditions, ranging from that of the badly crippled rheumatoid sufferer to that of the mild osteoarthritic. These exercises can even be used as an added benefit for patients who require hospital physiotherapy. Not all hospitals, private clubs and public facilities have pools but many of these exercises can be done at home in the bathtub.

Water exercises enable patients to assist in their own rehabilitation and spread their physical and spiritual wings to fly back to positive health, mobility and normality.

INTRODUCTION

The Arthritic's Book of Water Exercise has been written for anyone who has difficulty moving muscles or joints because of pain. Swimming ability is not necessary. Except for the clearly marked 'Advanced Exercises' in chapter 5, none of these movements require putting your face or head under the water. The only time you are required to lift both feet off the bottom of the pool simultaneously is when you are holding on to the edge of the pool securely, or when you are supported by a flotation device.

Although the main focus of our exercise programme is the chronic arthritis sufferer, this book is equally useful for those people who have undergone surgery, have had a severe accident that cannot be corrected by surgery, or have suffered impaired use of a limb or limbs because of a stroke. Any of these medical problems can cause severe pain and substantially limited movement. In all cases, the person who does not exercise affected muscles and joints has a good chance of losing the ability to move them through their full range of motion because the muscles will atrophy. The old adage 'move it or lose it' can be a literal prognosis. Following the programme outlined in this book can lead to a lifetime of satisfying activity, while ignoring it can contribute to unhappiness and crippling disability.

Unlike the other potential cripplers we have mentioned, arthritis is a progressive disease. Without medical treatment coupled with a programme of exercise, the sufferer can look forward to continuing pain and increasingly limited mobility of affected joints as he or she ages. Also, many forms of arthritis continue attacking new joints to limit overall body mobility as the disease progresses.

Unfortunately, at the present time, with 31.6 million arthritis sufferers in the USA and with 15 per cent of the population of the UK suffering from arthritis, *there is no known cure.* Only informed and knowledgeable management of the disease by the victim him- or herself can make a lasting difference in the amount of pain and the degree of permanent disability that is suffered. An arthritis-management programme must be undertaken with the guidance of a physician, supplemented by an approved regimen of rest and exercise.

This exercise programme was designed by Nancy Kadlec. After receiving her degree from the University of Iowa in 1965, she served as a registered occupational therapist for various governmental agencies including Hines V.A. Hospital, Alton State Hospital, and Madden Mental Health Center before joining the LaGrange, Illinois, YMCA aquatic staff in 1979. Judy Jetter, who received her BA in psychology from the University of Illinois, joined Nancy in 1980. Her original assignment was to teach adult swimming and general aquatic exercise, but her horizons were immediately broadened through her association with Nancy and her 'rusty hinges' programme, which served as the basis for the self-help programme described in this book. The man who appears in many of the photographs in this book is Bill Jetter, Judy's husband.

Nancy has worked closely with the Arthritis Foundation for many years, often lecturing to medical people as well as to those afflicted with the disease itself. Her programme of water exercise is recognized by the Arthritis Foundation, which has recently appointed her a member of their joint task force with the American YMCA organization to develop a standardized programme of exercise for people with motion impairments. In 1977 Nancy was diagnosed as having rheumatoid arthritis. The effects of her disease are painfully apparent in several of the close-up photographs of her hands, which clearly show the asymmetry of many of her fingers.

1
The Facts About Pain

Although anyone who suffers recurrent pain can use this book, it is aimed primarily at those who have undergone medical diagnosis and who have been advised by a physician to participate in a modified exercise programme. We strongly believe in the importance of checking with your doctor before you begin exercising to make sure that this programme is consistent with your overall medical treatment. Since we cannot attempt to answer detailed questions about your specific disease or recommended treatment, we urge you to take the time to acquaint yourself with the possible symptoms and the general progress to be expected of your particular illness. Our bibliography might be a good starting-point to discover this sort of information. Your doctor will give you specific advice about your individual condition. Don't be afraid to ask questions.

We've posed each picture to give you the clearest view of the particular exercise we describe. Often we have used two people, and sometimes three, to help you visualize the whole motion from beginning to end. The person on the left always begins the exercise and the one on the right holds the final position, to enable you to read the photograph the same way you read the words in the text, from left to right. Occasionally we have had to show a particular exercise out of the water so that you can get a clearer look at the correct body positioning. However, except for the isometric exercises shown in chapter 6, we don't recommend that you leave the water to do the exercises on land.

We have included a list of all the exercises in the Exercise Review Chart, on pages 115–25. There we indicate the specific joints or muscles benefited by each exercise, so that you can better concentrate on the places that hurt you. But remember, it is best to follow a well-rounded programme of exercise by doing at least the minimum number of repetitions of each exercise that we describe for your fitness level. (See chapter 2 for complete information and instructions.)

Sometimes the text also mentions the part of your body that will be affected if the particular exercise described causes a very strong feeling of pressure, stretching, or pulling. However, most of the movements described are designed to work on multiple muscles and joints simultaneously, so it is impractical to list each affected area of the body for each exercise. In other words, a gentle pull or stretch, even if it is not mentioned in the text, is all right. Of course, if a pulling or stretching feeling gives way to actual pain, the vigour with which you perform the exercise should be reduced, or the exercise should be eliminated entirely – at least temporarily.

Before you begin the programme we urge you to read the answers to questions we are asked most often about the exercises and their effect on various crippling disabilities. We think this will help you to understand our programme and how to use it.

Realistically speaking, what can I expect to gain from water exercise?

Further crippling or pain in affected joints will be slowed dramatically or arrested, even if your range of motion in some joints is very limited at the moment. Even more dramatic is the fact that the vast majority of people we have helped since this programme began have reported *increased* range of motion in affected joints. Some have even had their doctors reduce or eliminate medication prescribed for pain. Others have been able to walk unassisted by the crutches, canes, or walkers to which they believed they were tied for the rest of their lives.

These incredible results are not the product of imagination or magic. They are the body's natural response to a planned programme of gentle, controlled stretching and limbering movements emphasizing flexibility and joint mobility. Muscles are strengthened by the active resistance of the water itself, as the part of the body being exercised gently pushes against the weight of the water. This active motion is enhanced by the water's buoyancy, which minimizes the earth's gravitational pull on sore or deformed joints. Feelings of tension are soon replaced by a sense of relaxation because of the nature of the exercises themselves – particularly those geared for the shoulders and lower back. Gradually your body will build in strength and endurance. You will find that you can increase the duration and speed with which you perform each exercise. Naturally, these gains follow you out of the water and into your daily life. You will find that you can get more done before you become fatigued.

An added advantage to the water exercise programme is that while you are toning your muscles you will find your body becoming firmer and more attractive, no matter what your age. It generally takes a while for regular exercise to begin to bring about significant changes in body firmness, however, so don't be disappointed if you don't experience positive results immediately.

How will exercise relieve pain and immobility caused by accident or surgery?

Because the buoyancy of water overcomes gravity to a large degree, muscles and joints that have been damaged respond well to gentle stretching exercises done in water. Exercise therapy programmes are often prescribed for accident or surgery patients both in and out of the hospital. Your physician can tell you which exercises will be most helpful to your individual problem, but don't ignore the benefits you will get from following a gentle exercise programme for all areas of your body.

How will this programme help me if I have had a stroke?

To understand the effect exercise can have on paralysed muscles, first it is necessary to understand the nature of a stroke. When the blood supply that carries oxygen to the brain is interrupted, the result can be a sudden onset of symptoms such as weakness or paralysis on one side of the body coupled with visual, intellectual, or emotional disorders. The causes of this loss of oxygen to the brain are varied. Blood vessels and arteries in the brain may become blocked. Some blood vessels may be weakened, allowing blood to flow directly into the brain. If blood clots form, they can compress the material inside the brain, which causes damage.

Controlling diet and nervous tension, taking medication to control blood pressure, abstaining from smoking, and exercise therapy are just a few of the factors that will influence positively the outcome of a stroke.

It is important for family members to be aware that a stroke victim often experiences feelings of depression and anger, which interfere with the desire to be with others. Crowds and loud or constant noise may be very irritating. Stroke patients have very little energy and often try to avoid activity, which is unfortunate, since they also tend to experience feelings of isolation.

Exercise is of tremendous value to people who have had a stroke, because it prevents atrophy of affected muscles while it maintains or even increases the function of affected limbs. The whole body, in fact, is benefited by exercise, since it also improves circulation, respiration, and coordination. Therapeutic exercises are usually started while the patient is still in hospital and they generally take the form of physical or occupational therapy procedures. Unfortunately, exercise is often stopped when the patient returns home, because of lack of interest on the part of the patient or family, the considerable financial problems families often face, and sometimes the difficulty some people encounter in transporting themselves to the therapist.

Water exercise can be an answer to the patient's need to socialize, while he or she works to increase the range of motion of affected joints. Many municipalities have pools that are available at a small charge. Schools, health clubs, YMCA facilities, and hotels, although more expensive, can be used, too. Several patients who could afford it have had their own private pools installed in or out of doors. In the UK many of the larger hospitals have pools available for their arthritic patients under the National Health Service, and several private hospitals have pools also, in both cases with trained personnel in attendance.

Exactly what does medical science know about arthritis?

More than a hundred different types of arthritis affect people of both sexes, without regard to age, income, or the area in which they live. Dinosaur skeletons, as well as the remains of the earliest cave-dwellers, clearly show that this painful disease predates recorded history. For thousands of years people did not know what to do for the arthritis sufferer. Hundreds of remedies were tried, but none had more than limited success, including those devised by modern medicine. For many years doctors and those practising folk medicine said that arthritic joints should not be moved or exercised. Finally, within the last decade or two, the benefits of exercise have begun to be recognized. Unfortunately, exercise programmes for arthritics are often inadequate and don't allow sufferers to work up to their full potential because of the pain involved in exercising on land. Insufficient exercise causes further degeneration of the affected joints.

No cure has been found for this always painful and often crippling disease. Arthritis affects 31.6 million people in the

United States alone. It is the West's number-one crippling disease, and will affect one out of every seven people at some time in their lives.

Where is my arthritis likely to strike next? How painful can it get?

Depending upon the type and severity of your arthritis, the amount of exercise you regularly work into your daily life, your programme of weight control and general eating habits, and your own attitude towards your illness, you can have more or less control of your disease and its progressive symptoms. Although an in-depth discussion of each one of these factors cannot be covered in this book, we have included a brief bibliography for further reading and information. Here we are mainly concerned with the advantages of a well-defined exercise regime coupled with a sensible life-style.

In following the programme, regular pre-planned work periods with rest times in between are preferred. Do not make frantic attempts at tackling any complicated task, including this exercise programme. Instead, plan your activities and budget your time. You will find that you can relieve your own pain without resorting to increasing doses of painkillers. Arthritics who exercise regularly often report that they are able to cut back on medication prescribed for their pain. At the same time, they find that they enjoy a more active and unrestricted life than before they started exercising. Without such a programme of exercise and attention to rest and diet, they could only look forward to the painful progression of their disease.

It is impossible for us to list all the symptoms and facts about each type of arthritis, but we have highlighted information about the most common forms for easy reference. Remember, your doctor is always the best source for detailed information about your specific disease.

Rheumatoid arthritis generally strikes in the middle years of life, usually sometime after thirty. Three times as many women are affected as their male counterparts. Most often attacks are first experienced in the hands and feet. From there the disease generally travels to wrists, shoulders, and knees. Hips and ankles seem to be affected last. Symptoms include swelling and redness in joints. Fever is not uncommon. Rheumatoid arthritis is considered a chronic disease affecting the total body system.

Osteoarthritis usually occurs much later in life, at an average age of fifty-five. It begins at weight-bearing joints such as the spine, hips, knees, and ankles. From there it often moves to the ends of the fingers. Shoulder joints are the last to be affected. Osteoarthritis is a non-inflammatory form of arthritis which generally continues to attack the affected joint with increasing severity rather than travelling steadily throughout the entire body as does rheumatoid arthritis.

My doctor prescribes medicine for my pain so why should I exercise?

Your doctor prescribes medication to relieve your pain and to attempt to make you more comfortable. No reputable physician will prescribe unnecessary pain-relieving drugs, but since it is in the nature of the disease that your pain may progress and the number of painful joints may increase over a period of time, it is logical that your doctor may increase dosages or prescribe more and more potent drugs. Occasional pain flare-ups can boost the amount of medication required still further. Your doctor is well aware of the potential side effects of the drugs he prescribes, but he has no other alternative if you do not help by taking active responsibility for the control of your own disease. Although following some sort of exercise programme won't guarantee remission of your symptoms, exercise has been shown to be one of a combination of several important factors that can contribute to remission.

   Side effects caused by medication vary with the individual and the type and amount prescribed. A discussion of potential side effects is beyond the scope of this book, but your physician is the best source of information about the specifics of the medication he feels is best for you. Generally your doctor will begin with aspirin or paracetamol and move to more potent medication if your pain becomes more severe. Surgery is sometimes undertaken as a final resort to correct or prevent deformities and to ease pain and stabilize a particular joint, allowing it to function more fully.

This aquatic exercise programme is designed to keep your joints limber enough so that substantial dosages or the use of increasingly sophisticated pain-relievers can be deferred. People who stick to this programme usually report actually needing less of whatever drug they generally take.

2
Getting Down to Specifics

The water exercises in this book have been developed by a registered occupational therapist. They have been tested on hundreds of patients. However, this programme is not meant to replace the recommendations of your personal physicians, but only to supplement them.

Why will water exercise help me feel better?

Water is an ideal medium for relieving pain and stiffness in muscles and joints. Because your body is almost weightless in water, the range of motion you can perform in an affected joint is considerably greater than on dry land. On the other hand, water also offers resistance to help build muscle strength and tone.

Each person has a slightly different optimum comfort level related to water temperature, but the comfort range for most people falls between 78 °F and 85 °F (25.5–29.5 °C). As a general rule, the more vigorous your exercise, the cooler you will want the water.

Most arthritis sufferers are concerned mainly about the painful joints they feel at the moment. They are apt to neglect those joints they believe to be 'healthy'. This is a mistake, since your general body tone must be maintained. Of course, when major flare-ups occur, your doctor may suggest that you cut back or even skip your exercise sessions for a while. Just be sure the interruptions don't become permanent. Our programme is designed to provide exercise for all the major muscle groups and joints, and it can be used by arthritis sufferers and anyone else who has pain, even if movement is severely impaired. See the chart on pages 115–25 for exercises for specific areas of pain. The number of repetitions necessary for each exercise is dependent on your general physical condition and the specific areas of your body that are affected.

How often and how long should I exercise each time?

The amount of time spent on an individual session, as well as the number of sessions each week, depends entirely on your doctor's recommendations, which are in turn related to your individual condition and the availability of a pool or lake. We have included a section of exercises that can be done in the bath to enable you to supplement your regular programme when necessary.

If you are just starting your programme of exercise, five short sessions of perhaps fifteen minutes each for a week or so are ideal to limber your joints without causing fatigue, which could cancel out the positive benefits. You can then gradually decrease the number of sessions to two or three a week, while you simultaneously increase the amount of time you spend at each session to a maximum of forty-five minutes.

We realize that not everyone will be able to follow this ideal regimen. But remember, some exercise is better than none. Visit the water as often as you can, even if it is only a couple of times each week. Don't give up if you miss a few sessions, either. After all, you can still work out in the bath. (See chapter 7 and the asterisked exercises in the other chapters that you can include in your bath workout.)

How do I know if the exercises are too easy or too difficult?

Since the first set of 'Beginner Exercises' is also used as a warm-up for every subsequent series, everyone starts from the same point, no matter what the level of each person's physical condition. Some people will stay at the beginner level for many weeks before moving on to the 'Beginner Plus' exercises. Others with less motion impairment will breeze through the first few series and quickly settle down to water bicycling and waist twists. Until you can do the maximum number of repetitions of a particular exercise set without fatigue or pain, it is best not to move on to those that are more difficult.

The 'Advanced Exercises' are for swimmers only. These exercises are best performed in deep water, although some are suited to the shallow end of the pool, provided that you are comfortable and can maintain stable equilibrium with both feet off the ground simultaneously. Don't worry if you can't work up to this part of the programme. Every muscle and joint used in the 'Advanced Exercises' will have already gone through an excellent workout in the less vigorous exercises.

It is important to do as much as you can, but don't work past your own individual point of genuine pain or fatigue. If time permits after you finish the first set of exercises, go on to the next, again doing each exercise in turn. It is only necessary to do the minimum number of repetitions of any exercise if the exercise does not address your particular areas of pain. Concentrate on doing more repetitions of those that pertain to your specific problem areas.

How will I know if I am doing enough exercise, or if I am doing too much?

Your own body will tell you how much exercise you should do if only you will listen to it. Many people can do no more than fifteen minutes of exercise when they begin the programme. Others can start with the full forty-five-minute recommended time for each session. Some people must rest every few minutes, while others can breeze through the whole series from beginning to end without a break. A few even swim after the exercise session is over.

The trick is always to recognize your limitations, but to increase your total exercise time and the number of repetitions you do during each session. Your progress must be gradual but steady, unless you are having a temporary flare-up. Rheumatoid flare-ups are characterized by multiple red, hot, swollen joints. Notify your doctor if these symptoms occur. He or she may suggest that you shorten your exercise sessions, avoid becoming chilled, or omit your exercises for a while.

If you find that you cannot increase your total exercise time or the number of repetitions you do during each session, it is probably time for another visit to your physician. But remember, the key words are *gradual* and *steady*. Your end gain will be zero if you wear yourself out at your first session or two and then give up.

I'm a pretty good swimmer. Why don't I just swim steady lengths?

Swimming is the best of all exercises if you're up to it. We encourage everyone to include it in an overall exercise programme. But don't make the mistake of limiting your exercise to swimming. Sometimes certain joints are neglected in a swimming regimen, since often the swimmer doesn't know how to do more than one or two different strokes. Then, too, some strokes are impossible to do, even if you know how, because they cause severe pain in a particular joint or even in several joints. Our programme has been designed to utilize all the potentially affected joints in as full a range of motion as possible without straining them to the point of damage.

Where can I go to exercise?

The first choice for any programme of water exercise is a swimming pool rather than the sea. Water depth and bottom conditions are clearly marked and visible. Waves and undertows pose no problems, and you can use the sides of the pool for support when necessary. The walls and sides are also exercise tools.

Some areas of the country have a local YMCA and there are more and more health clubs opening, though many of us can't afford the hefty membership fees charged by private clubs.

If you prefer to exercise in an open body of water, be sure it is properly patrolled, especially if you are not a very good swimmer, and be sure the water is not too chilly. Find at least one other person to exercise with so that you can keep an eye on each other. You will find that it is more fun to exercise with a friend, and even better to get a small group together, if you can. But the water must be warm.

Can I exercise at home?

Chapters 6 and 7 are valuable when it is not convenient to visit a swimming pool, or even when you have a really painful flare-up. They describe exercises that can be done at home in your bath, and include isometric exercises that won't cause additional pain in the already sore areas of your body. In addition, we have marked with an asterisk all the exercises in the preceding chapters that can also be done at home in a full bath. Remember, however, that at-home exercises are only for temporary situations. They will not replace the total exercise programme designed for the pool.

Have you any tips on buying a bathing suit?

No one brand of swimsuit is better than another, and price is a very poor gauge of quality. Nancy usually selects a traditional type of suit (*left*), while Judy generally swims in the inexpensive body-suit pictured here.

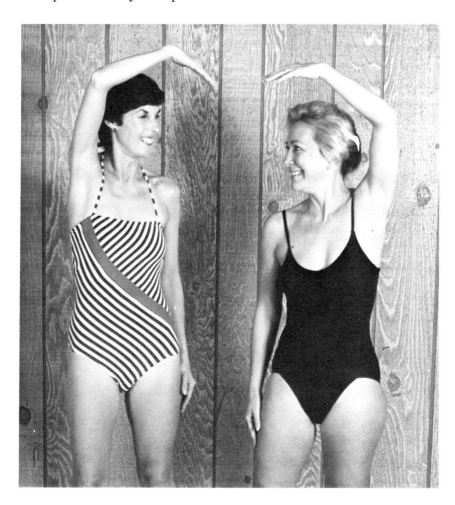

It is probably best to begin your water exercises with the suit you now own, as long as it fits properly and is comfortable and easy to slip into. If you feel that you look good in a particular style or colour, by all means wear it, even if it does not conform to our suggestions. A positive attitude is going to be a tremendous help in the overall effectiveness of your exercise programme, and you should do everything you can to reinforce it.

When you do get ready to shop for a new swimsuit, you may want to consider some of these factors. Sanforized cotton, although still quite acceptable (particularly in men's fashions) has been replaced for the most part by nylon or Lycra blends. When new, the Lycra tends to mould to your body more easily than nylon. It is also generally easier to put on and take off than nylon. However, it does not wear nearly as well as nylon and has a marked tendency to bag and stretch after a while. Chlorine and other chemical additives commonly used to disinfect and condition pool water can cause either material to fade, but Lycra fibres are more vulnerable to these chemicals. No matter what your preference in fabrics, remember that a wet suit sometimes seems to have a mind of its own, and a wise buyer takes ease of dressing and undressing into consideration.

Men may wear either boxer or brief-type trunks, as long as the elastic doesn't bind around the waist or legs. You will probably want to avoid solid shades of white, tan, or brown. White trunks tend to become transparent when wet, and the others can give the impression of nudity from a distance.

One-piece suits are preferred by most women, more from a comfort standpoint than out of consideration for style or body type. Make sure the straps are reasonably wide and set close to the neck. Criss-crossed straps in the back add security. If your suit has wide-set shoulder straps you can ask someone to tie them together with a shoelace or a piece of string close to your shoulder blades to keep them from falling off your shoulders while you exercise. Swimsuits with foam padding in the bra or with extra material forming a skirt tend to add to your buoyancy in the water, making your footing less secure. This is not the type of suit for you if you are a poor swimmer.

Those who have had a mastectomy will find that special swimsuits are available at better stores. However, the added buoyancy factor may make a poor swimmer unsure of her footing in water at chest level or above. A simple, dark-coloured, unpadded suit is probably a better choice.

Some people are concerned about modesty and may be tempted to give up on water exercise simply because of inadequate privacy in the dressing rooms. Nancy models a simple, inexpensive cover-up made from a single beach towel, which she designed. It will keep you warm while going to and from the pool area, can be used as a towel, and can be kept on while dressing or undressing unless you need to slip something over your head.

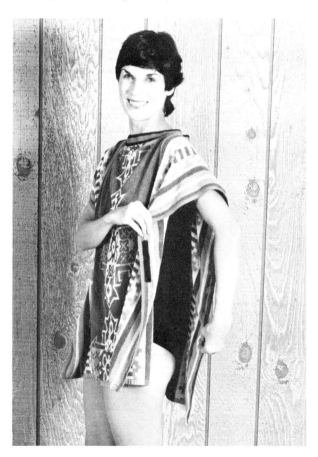

Pool Cover-up Instructions

You'll need a beach towel, two sets of colour-coordinated Velcro strips, and needle and thread to make this inexpensive cover-up.

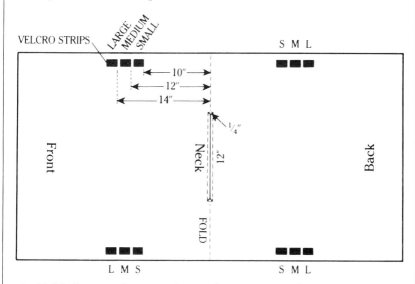

1. Fold the towel crosswise and cut a 12-inch opening in the centre along the fold. Make the opening a little bigger if your hairstyle is full.
2. Clip the corners of the opening $\frac{1}{4}$ inch so that the neck will lie flat. Turn material under and stitch round the entire opening.
3. Measure 10 inches down from the neck opening if you wear a size small, 12 inches if you are a medium, and 14 inches if you generally buy a large, and sew the Velcro strips down each side, front and back, from that point. This will form the armholes.

Be sure to close the Velcro strips when you wash your cover-up in a machine so that they don't snag other garments.

Do I need any special kind of equipment?

Most of these exercises are done without special equipment, but minibike-size inner tubes are probably the best buy if you plan to tackle the 'Intermediate Plus' and 'Advanced Exercises'. They can be bought at most bike shops. Be sure to tape the air valve securely with electrical tape to prevent it from scratching your skin. The small plastic tubes sold in toy shops are okay, too, but as you get stronger you may very well find that they don't hold enough air to offer the best resistance or buoyancy.

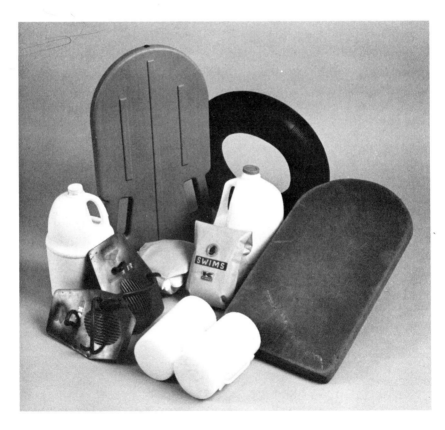

Clockwise from top: Inner tube, kickboard, pull buoys, hand paddles, detergent bottle, kickboard with hand grips
Centre: Plastic container, arm floats

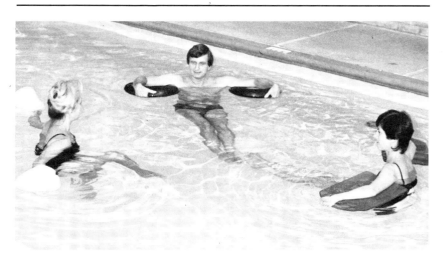

If you would rather use a Styrofoam kickboard you can pick one up at most sports shops. An inexpensive substitute for a tube or kickboard can be found in your laundry cupboard or refrigerator. An empty plastic gallon detergent container is quite effective. Just be sure the handle is wide enough for comfort, especially if you have pain in your wrists or fingers.

Painful or stiff shoulder joints should always be treated gently. Don't hang on to the sides of the pool, but use two of the floating devices we have described above. Small inflatable plastic wrist and ankle bands can be purchased in any toy shop, and when slipped over wrists or ankles will add resistance during your water exercises. Don't rely on them to hold you up, though.

Final tips before beginning your exercises

Pain is nature's way of telling you that you may be doing too much and should cut back or stop a particular exercise or exercise set. *Don't continue with any exercise that causes pain unless your doctor specifically advises you to.* Arthritis sufferers in particular must be aware that further damage to a muscle or joint can occur if pain is ignored. Don't fall into the trap of believing your ability to withstand pain while exercising is going to help you feel better later on. It won't. Instead, you may cause yourself a setback or even suffer greater injury and more pain.

When performing these exercises keep your back straight and hold in your stomach muscles. To avoid neck injury, never tilt your head backwards at a severe angle. Your eyes should be open at all times to help maintain your balance. Always begin each session with the beginner warm-up exercises. Don't skip this important first step when you have progressed up to the second or third level – a warm-up period is still necessary. Finally, remember to breathe regularly. Don't hold your breath for any reason. None of these exercises requires putting your face in the water.

You'll have a lot more fun if you can arrange to exercise with a friend, or even get a small group together. People stimulate each other by offering both practical help and psychological support. Friends will take an awful lot of the work out of each session while putting enjoyment into it, so don't hesitate to phone a couple of your friends and ask them to join you. If that fails, do it by yourself anyway. You may encounter someone at the pool who, seeing what you are doing, asks to join in.

3
Beginner Exercises

Each person beginning this exercise programme has a different level of stamina based not only on his or her overall physical fitness level, but on the type and progress of his or her particular illness. Therefore, you should consult your doctor before beginning this or any other exercise programme.

If you are having a lot of pain or are experiencing a painful flare-up, or if you haven't exercised for many years, begin with a minimum number of four repetitions for each of these 'Beginner Exercises' with the exception of the first six. Gradually move on to six repetitions of each exercise, working towards an eventual eight, or even more if you find a particular exercise very beneficial. Stick to this first section until you can move at a steady pace through a maximum of eight repetitions each for the whole series without becoming too fatigued. At this point you can safely move on to the 'Intermediate Exercises', using these as a warm-up series.

As you look at the photographs you will occasionally notice minor deviations in body positions, particularly in the width of the stance, angle of an arm or leg, or the height to which it is raised. For example, generally Nancy's feet are wider apart than Judy's. This results from individual differences in flexibility and general physical condition, as well as minor differences in height and in body proportions. You must also take your own individual body type and condition into consideration when performing these exercises. Strive to get maximum motion as long as you don't push yourself past your physical limitations or your own specific level of pain.

If no specific mention is made of hand or foot placement in a particular exercise, just do whatever feels most comfortable to you. People who have experienced stiff or painful fingers are advised to grasp the pool edge gently, or to drape their wrists over the side of the pool or other steadying device rather than to grip it forcefully. If you have never had problems with your fingers then the possibility of causing any harm is lessened.

NOTE *Exercises that can be done in a bath are marked with asterisks.*

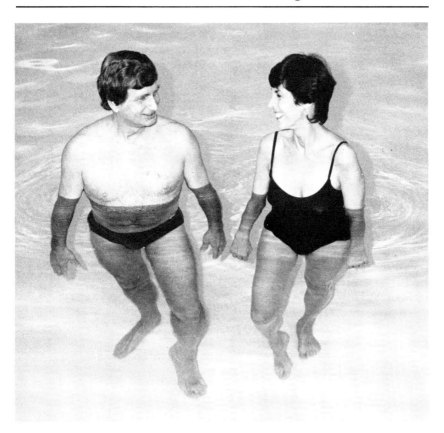

1. STICKY STRUT

Spread your feet so they are about 3 inches apart, hands at your
sides. Hands may swing naturally if you are more comfortable
this way. Pretend that you have something sticky on the balls of
your feet while you try to walk. Because your toes are stuck to
the ground you can only lift your heels. Continue shifting your
weight, making sure to keep your back straight and your chin
high. Repeat as rapidly as you can for a minute or two.

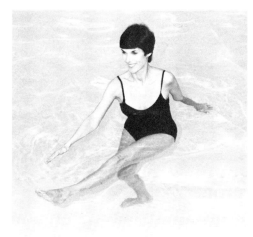

2. STRAIGHT-LEG MARCH

Stretch your arms out to the side for balance while you walk forward lifting each leg as high as you can without straining. The knee of your raised leg should be held straight. Point the toes of your raised foot at the ceiling. Walk as briskly as possible for at least six steps. Gradually increase the number of steps you take until you can maintain this march for several minutes. For added benefit, as pictured, extend the arm opposite your lifted leg. Try to touch your toe, but be sure to keep your back straight. You may feel a pulling sensation in the back of your extended leg.

CAUTION *Omit the toe touch if you suffer from backaches.*

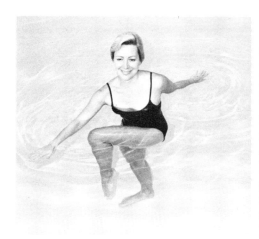

3. BENT-LEG MARCH

This is similar to the straight-leg march, but this time bend your knee as high as you can when your foot comes off the floor. Point the toes of your raised leg downwards. Don't extend your leg forwards at all. Begin with six steps and gradually work up to several minutes. For added benefit, extend the arm opposite your lifted knee with each step.

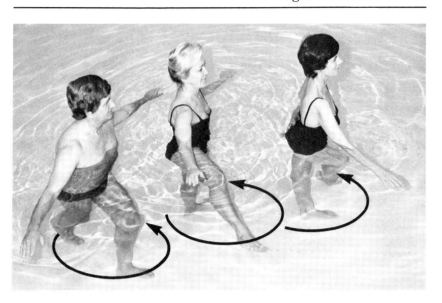

4. SEMI-CIRCLE STRUT

Your arms are extended to the side. Your weight is on your left leg. Keeping your right knee as straight as possible, swing your right leg in a large semi-circle in front of your left leg. Put your right foot down and shift your weight on to that leg. Now swing your left leg out, cross it in front of your right foot, and set it down. Repeat. After a few minutes, when you feel confident of your balance, semi-circle strut backwards by placing one foot behind the other. Keep your back straight throughout. You may feel a sensation in your hip or groin as you swing your leg.

CAUTION *People with artificial hips should not cross one leg in front of the other. Be sure your leg swings only to the centre of your body.*

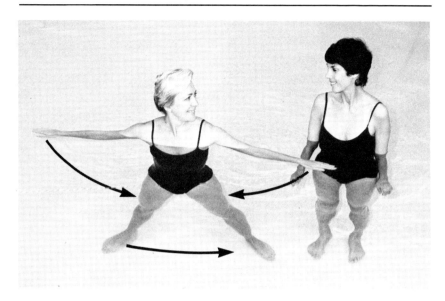

5. SIDE-STEP SHUFFLE

While your arms are extended to the side, stretch your left leg sideways as far as you can comfortably. Slide your right foot up to the left foot and set it down. Shift your weight back to the right foot and repeat the sideways movement with your left foot. You will move in the same direction with each step until you reverse direction by extending your right foot to the right, bringing your left foot up to it. Do the same number of repetitions in both directions. You may feel a stretch in the groin area of your extended leg.

    For added benefit bring your hands down to your thighs as the second foot closes the gap. Then extend your arms to the side, shoulder-high, as the first foot begins the movement over again. This is a very graceful arm motion, similar to a bird in flight. You may feel a stretching sensation in your shoulders.

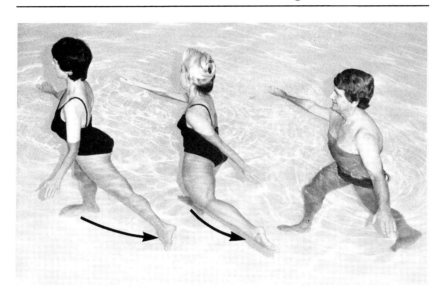

6. BACKWARDS WALK

With your arms extended, put your left leg behind you, bending
your knees slightly, if necessary. Land on the ball of your foot
and roll your foot backwards until it is flat on the ground.
Continue walking backwards, this time extending your right leg
behind you. Be sure to keep your back straight and lift your leg
from the hip. Hips and feet are the two areas most affected by
this exercise.

   For even greater benefit, lift the arm opposite the active leg,
as pictured, as high as you can as you step backwards. (Your
right arm moves straight upwards as your left foot swings
backwards; then your left arm moves straight upwards as your
right foot swings behind you.) Continue for a minute or two. You
may feel this arm motion in your shoulders.

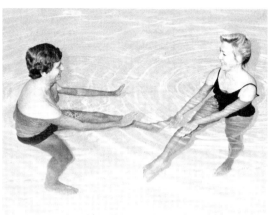

7. WAVE AT THE FISHES*

Lift your foot off the bottom and wave it up and down from the ankle, pointing and extending your toes. At the same time, wave your hands up and down from the wrist. Keep your back straight and your head up. Repeat with your right foot.

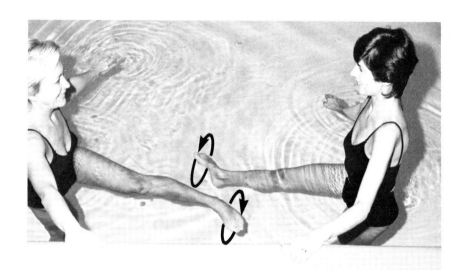

8. ANKLE CIRCLES*

Stand straight with your head up and your profile to the wall. Steady yourself by placing your right hand on the edge of the pool. Raise your left leg and circle your foot from the ankle only, then reverse the motion as if you are unwinding it. Turn to the other side and repeat with the right foot.

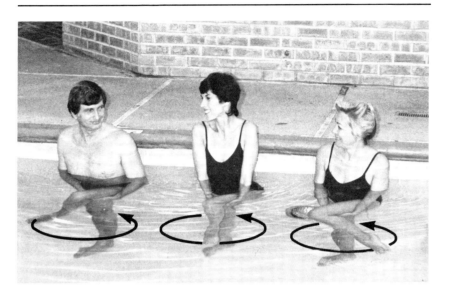

9. CAN-CAN

Brace yourself against the wall and support your left knee by grasping both hands under your left thigh. Now move your lower leg in a circle from your knee joint, first in one direction and then in the other. Change to the other leg and repeat the circles. Keep your back straight. You may feel a sensation in your knee.

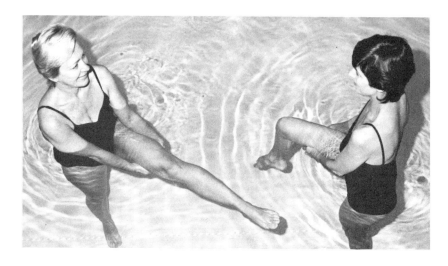

10. KNEE ROCK

Your hands support one knee under the thigh. Lift your straight leg forward as you point your toes to the ceiling. Then relax your toes and bend your leg under your thigh as far as you can. Keep your back straight and your chin level. You are likely to feel a stretch in the back of the active leg. Continue. Switch to the other leg.

11. STRAIGHT-LEG SWING/FRONT TO BACK

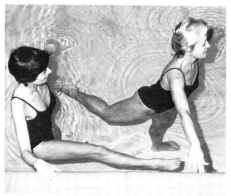

Stand with the right side of your body near the pool edge as you stabilize yourself with your right hand. Extend your left hand to the side for additional balance. With your toes pointed, swing your right leg forwards and backwards as far as is comfortable. Try not to bend your knee any more than is absolutely necessary to avoid pain. Keep your back straight and your chin level. You may feel a pulling in your swinging leg and hip. Turn round and repeat with your left leg.

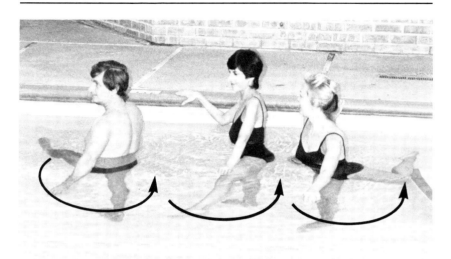

12. LEG ARC

Stabilize yourself with your right hand on the pool edge, left arm outstretched to the side. Lift your left leg as high as you can in front of you. Make a horizontal arc round the side, ending behind your body as far as it can go. You may allow your knee to bend as your leg approaches its extreme rear position. Be sure your back is straight and your chin is level. Now swing your leg round to the front. Repeat. Reverse position (left hand on the pool edge) and change to the other leg.

CAUTION *People with artificial hips should not cross one leg in front of the other. Be sure your leg swings only to the centre of your body.*

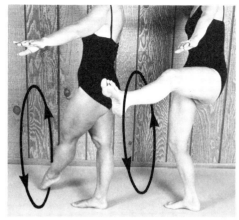

13. LEG CIRCLES

Stand with your right side comfortably away from the pool edge. You may extend your left hand to the side for additional stability. Brace your body with your right hand on the edge of the pool and swing your left leg in a wide vertical circle, making sure to keep your knee as straight as possible, although it may bend a little. Your hip does all the work. Continue. Now reverse your circle. Turn round and repeat with your right leg. You may feel a pulling sensation on the inside of your thigh.

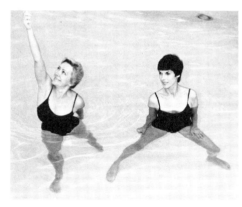

14. MONEY TREE

Imagine a tree with ten-pound notes for leaves and diamonds for flowers. Now reach up with your right arm and pick your fortune off the branches. Your left hand remains at your side. It is fine to put most of your weight on your right leg while the left leg stabilizes your balance. Be sure to look at your outstretched hand so that you see what you are picking from the tree. Put your 'fortune' into your 'side pocket' by bending your right elbow as you lower your hand parallel to your body. Repeat with your left hand. You will feel a gentle stretch in your chest as you raise your arm.

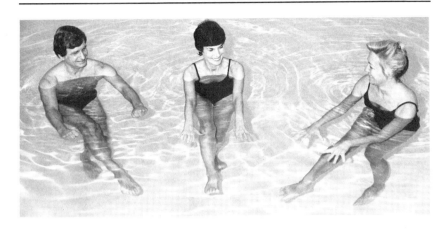

15. CURLY FINGERS AND TOES*

Make a fist with both hands and curl the toes of your slightly raised right foot. Now straighten out your fingers and toes. Finally, spread them. Repeat the same sequence with both hands and your left foot. You may want to brace your back against the pool wall if you feel you need to stabilize your balance. Remember to keep your head up. Repeat.

16. WEIGHTED THUMBS*

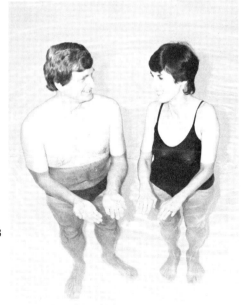

Keep your elbows tucked tightly against your sides. Extend your forearms so they are parallel to the pool bottom, palms facing upwards. Rotate your palms 180° so they face directly downwards. Rotate them again in the opposite direction until they face up again. Repeat. If you imagine you have a small weight attached to each thumb it will remind you to rotate your hands further in each direction. You will feel a twisting in your elbows and forearms.

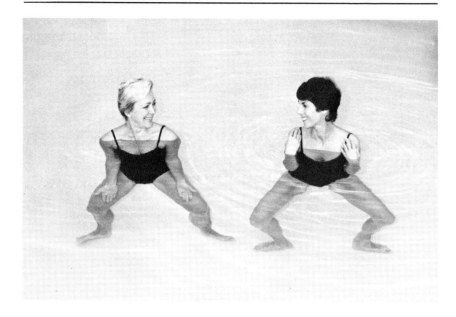

17. ELBOW BEND*

Spread your feet wide enough apart to maintain your balance.
Lower your body by bending at your knees, keeping your back
straight, until your shoulders are near or in the water. Tuck
your elbows into your waist, palms upwards, backs of your
hands against your thighs. Now imagine that you are lifting the
water up as you bend your elbows and raise your hands in front
of your body, until your fingers touch your shoulders. Lower
your forearms, making sure that your elbows are still tucked
into your waist, until your hands brush your thighs. Repeat.

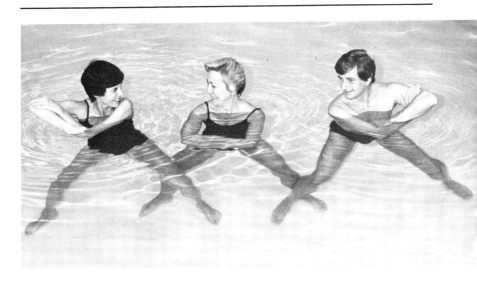

18. ROCKING THE BABY*

Place each hand on or near the opposite elbow. Spread your feet
wide apart in order to stabilize yourself and to allow your
shoulders to dip near or into the water. In this position raise
your arms to the right as far as you can. Your right elbow will be
high in the air and out of the water. Reverse the arc, brushing
your body with your upper arms as they pass in front of you.
Now swing your arms to the left as far as they will go, left elbow
high. You may feel a stretch in your chest and shoulders as you
raise each elbow.

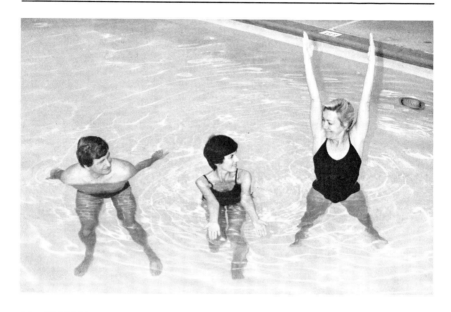

19. VICTORY

Spread your feet apart about shoulder width so that you have a good base of support. Breathe in and bend both knees as you lift your arms straight back behind you. Exhale as you swing your arms forward and up until they are straight over your head. Elbows should not be bent. Your knees will straighten naturally as you lift forward and up. As your arms swing overhead, rise up on your toes. Swing down to the starting position and repeat. You will feel a gentle stretch throughout your whole body.

CAUTION *People with heart problems must be aware of the extra stress on the heart during this exercise. Omit it if you experience any pain or dizziness, or at your physician's recommendation.*

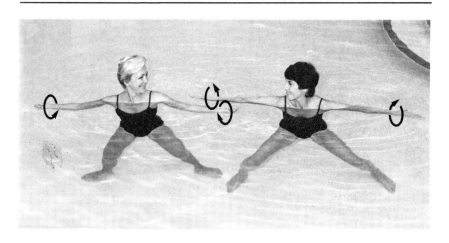

20. SHOULDER ROLL

Spread your feet apart and bend your knees until your shoulders
reach the water. Keep your back straight. Stretch your arms
straight out to the side, about shoulder height, palms to the
ceiling. Now clench your fists. Rotate your palms downwards
and all the way round, gradually opening your fists until your
palms are again facing the ceiling. Be sure the rolling motion
comes from your shoulders down to your hands. Return to the
starting position and repeat.

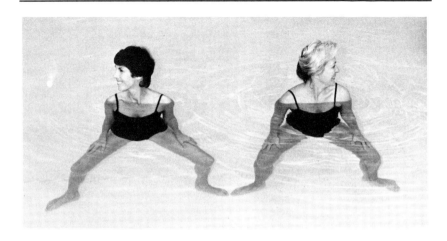

21. SIDE GLANCE*

With your feet spread comfortably apart, bend your knees until your shoulders are near the water. Keep your back straight. You may want to put your hands on your thighs for added balance. Now turn your head to the right as far as you can and find a landmark point as far as possible to the extreme right of your field of vision. Rotate your head slowly to the left and try to spot the same landmark point. Be sure to keep your shoulders perfectly straight and still so that your head turns from the neck only. You may feel a stretch in your neck opposite to the way your head is turned.

CAUTION *Because some necks are very delicate, we strongly recommend that your doctor be advised before you do this exercise.*

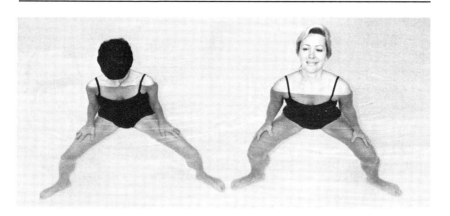

22. YES, YES*

With your feet spread comfortably apart, knees bent, lower your chin to your chest, then raise it until you are looking straight ahead. Don't shift your chin high in the air. It should be parallel to the bottom of the pool. You may feel a stretching in the back of your neck when your chin is lowered. Put your hands on your thighs for extra balance.

CAUTION *Because some necks are very delicate, we strongly recommend that your doctor be advised before you do this exercise.*

23. PICTURE FRAME*

Grasp each elbow with the opposite hand as you bend your knees. Raise your bent arms up and over your head. Try to get them high enough to pass your ears, if you can. Hold this position for a second or two before you lower your arms. Repeat. You may feel a stretching in your shoulders, elbows, and chest.

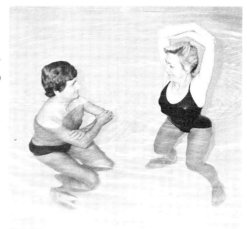

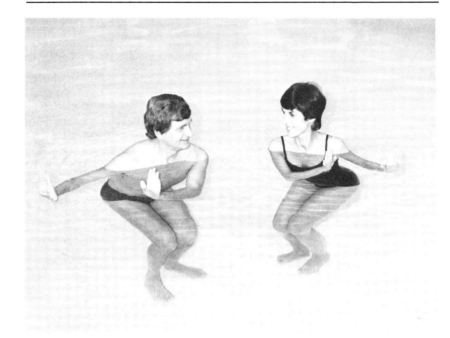

24. CHARLESTON

Stand with your knees slightly bent, toes of both feet pointing left, elbows flexed, and fingers pointing upwards. Face your palms outwards, to the right of your body. Pivot on your heels and swing your toes to the right as your arms swing to the left. Now pivot on your toes while you swing your heels to the right, swinging your arms back to the right at the same time. You will be moving in a sideways direction to the right. Repeat for 4 feet, then reverse direction and return to where you started. You may feel pressure on your knees or on the soles of your feet. Discontinue this exercise if the movement becomes uncomfortable.

25. PUSH, LIFT, BEND, AND STRETCH (Illustration p. 42)

Grasp a small inner tube or board, or any other buoyant object of similar size, making sure that your hands are on the opposite sides. Bend your elbows to raise it to your chest. It will be vertical at this point. Straighten your elbows to raise it horizontally over your head. Bend your elbows to lower it vertically behind your head. Return it to the straight-up, horizontal position. Lower it vertically in front of your chest again. Finally, push it horizontally down into the water. Repeat the whole sequence. You may feel this exercise in your shoulders, upper arms, elbows, hands and chest.

CAUTION *People with heart problems must be aware of the extra stress on the heart during this exercise. Omit it if you experience any pain or dizziness, or at your physician's recommendation.*

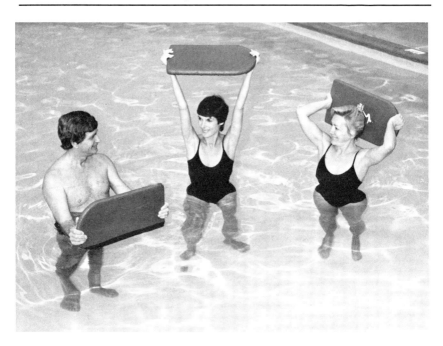

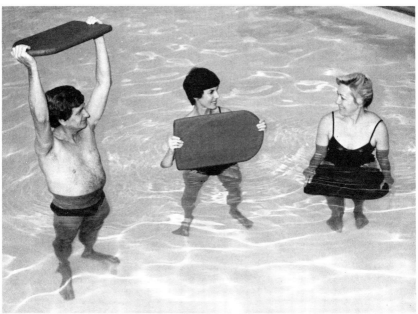

Beginner Plus

These movements are a bit more difficult to perform than the preceding exercises. Do not attempt them until you can do the 'Beginner Exercises' at least the suggested minimum number of repetitions without excessive strain.

Some may have to work into the following exercises more gradually by doing fewer repetitions the first few times. Don't give up! *You will soon work up to the full number as you build strength and stamina.*

26. KNEE-UP*

With your right side near the wall stabilize yourself with your right hand on the pool edge. Grasp your bent left knee and bring it up to your nose. Your shoulders will move forward naturally and the middle of your back will round out. Repeat. Turn round and do the same thing with your right knee.

CAUTION *Do not pull your knee towards you if you have an artificial hip or knee.*

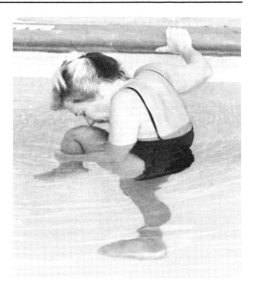

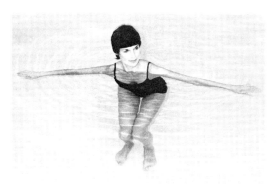

27. KNEE SQUATS

Point your feet forward, knees together. Spread your feet comfortably apart (at least several inches) for better stability. Arms are outstretched to each side. Bend your knees as far as you can comfortably, while keeping your heels on the floor. Then straighten up. Try to keep your back straight. Movements must be smooth and relatively slow. Repeat. You may feel a stretch in your calves.

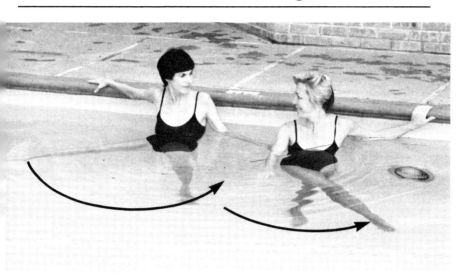

28. TICK-TOCK SWING

Brace your back against the side of the pool as you face forwards.
You may want to hold the pool edge with one arm for more
stability. With your weight on your left leg, swing your right leg
to the left in an arc, keeping it close to your body. Be sure to keep
your leg straight. Now swing it back to the right as far as you
can. This motion will be as smooth as the arc of a clock's
pendulum. Repeat this exercise with your left leg. You may feel
a stretch on the inside of your thigh as you swing your leg.

CAUTION *If you have an artificial hip do not cross that leg in front
of the other. Swing your leg* only *to the centre of your body.*

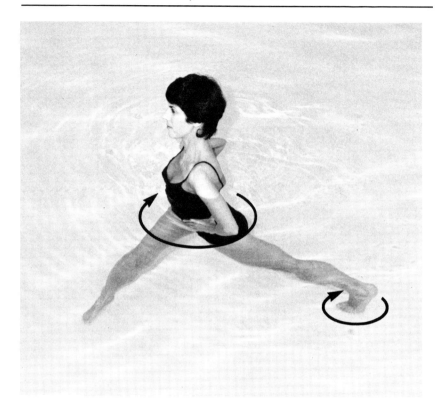

29. WAIST TWIST

Face front with your feet comfortably wide apart, hands on hips. Twist to the right, pivoting on the ball of your left foot as shown in the photo. Then twist to the other side, pivoting on the ball of your right foot. You will feel the twist in your torso and back.

CAUTION *If you have a bad back or if you experience any pain in your back while doing this exercise, twist less or omit the exercise entirely.*

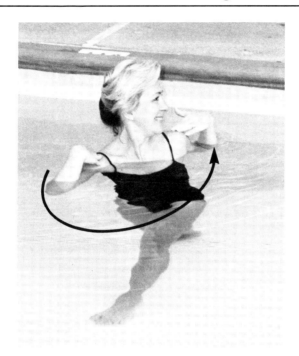

30. AGITATOR

Your feet must be comfortably apart, one in front of the other.
Bend your knees until your shoulders are in or near the water.
Touch your shoulders with your fingertips, lifting your elbows
up until your upper arms are parallel to the bottom of the pool.
Now twist your body as far as you can to the left and then to the
right. Let your head turn with your body. Try to find one central
point behind you that you can spot as you twist to each side. Be
sure your back remains straight. (An added benefit of this
agitator-like motion is the lovely elbow massage created by the
action of the swirling water.) You will feel a stretch in your
chest and back.

CAUTION *If you have a bad back or if you experience any pain in
your back while doing this exercise, twist less or omit the exercise
entirely.*

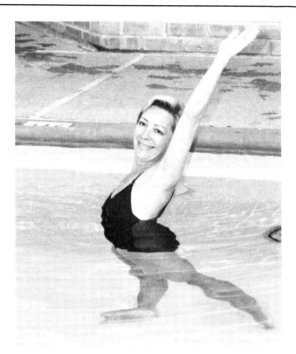

31. SUPER STRETCH

With your side to the pool wall, stand about an arm's length away and stabilize yourself with your right hand on the pool edge. Lift your left arm straight overhead while you kick backwards with your left leg. Point your toes. Be sure your elbow and knee remain straight. Alternate left and right sides. You may feel a stretch in your mid- or lower back and chest.

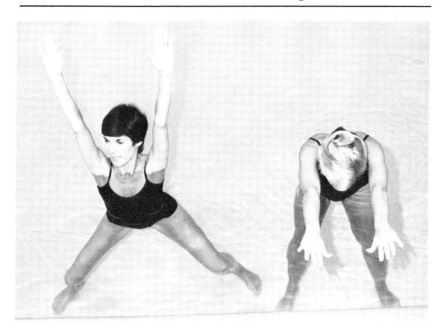

32. TAKE A BOW

Facing the pool wall, an arm's length from the edge, begin with
your arms raised directly overhead, elbows straight, chin
parallel to the pool bottom. Your legs should be spaced
comfortably apart. Be sure to tuck in your stomach muscles.
Now bend your upper body slowly forward from the waist until
you touch the edge of the pool with your fingertips. Your knees
may be slightly flexed for comfort. Repeat. You will feel a
stretch in your back and shoulders and a contraction in your
waist and abdomen.

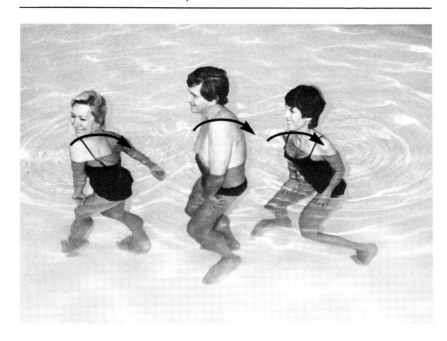

33. MAE WEST*

With your feet comfortably apart at about shoulder width, bend
your knees until your shoulders are near the water. Keep your
chin level and your stomach muscles tucked in. Rotate your left
shoulder in a circular motion, front to back, lifting it as high as
you are able. Do the usual number of repetitions and then switch
to your right shoulder. Repeat, reversing the motion of each
shoulder (back to front). It is not essential to keep your fingers
on your thighs.

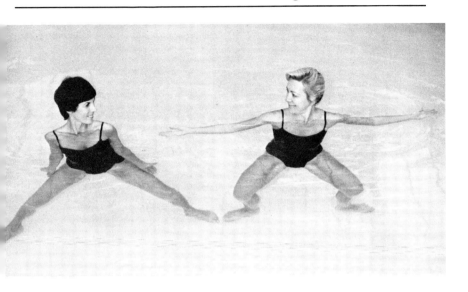

34. SIDE ARM LIFT

Stand with feet apart. Bend your knees until your chin nears the
water. Arms are at your sides, the little finger of each hand
brushing your thighs. Lift your arms upwards to shoulder
height, elbows straight, palms up. Don't bring your arms
forward. Return to starting position and repeat. You may feel
water resistance on your shoulders.

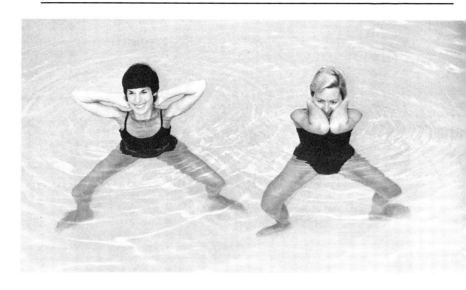

35. ELBOW KISS

Stand straight, knees slightly bent, feet comfortably apart, fingers loosely interlaced behind your head. Inhale as you bring your elbows forward until they are as close together as possible, touching if you can. Now swing them backwards naturally as far as you are able as you exhale. Your hands will force your neck to move forward slightly. Counter this motion by pushing backwards with your head. Remember to keep your tummy muscles tight. This exercise works the muscles in your upper back as well as your shoulders.

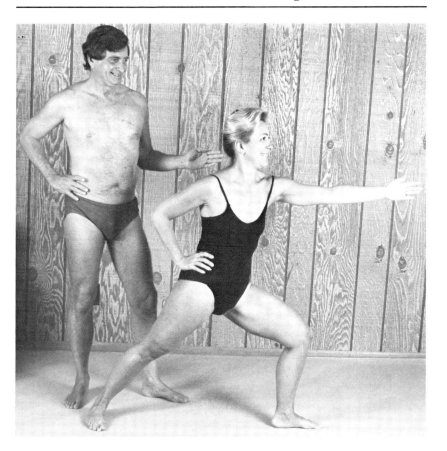

36. FENCING

Put your right hand on your hip. Your feet are comfortably apart,
toes pointed to the front. Turn your left foot to the left and lunge
forward over your left foot, bending your knee and thrusting
your left arm until it's straight. Your right foot should not move.
The motion resembles a sword fighter's movements. Repeat.
Switch to your right side. You may feel pressure on your bent
knee and a stretch in your extended arm and shoulder.

4
Intermediate Exercises

Don't tackle this section until you are comfortable doing the 'Beginner Exercises' at least eight times each. Then continue to use the beginner series as a warm-up. Remember, if you encounter any pain decrease the range of your motion so that you are not reaching or stretching so much, or do the exercise less vigorously. You may even choose to omit it for a while.

NOTE *Exercises that can be done in a bath are marked with asterisks.*

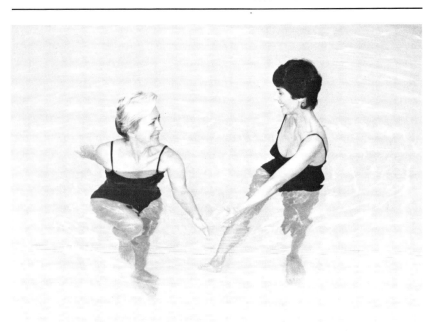

37. KICK WALK

Begin by bending your right knee while you swing your straight left arm forward. Relaxed toes point downwards. Now stretch your leg forward by straightening your knee as you point your toes upwards. Return your foot to the floor as your leg remains straight. Be sure to land on the ball of your foot. Alternate left and right legs, remembering to swing the opposite straight arm forward simultaneously. The effect will be primarily on your knees and hips.

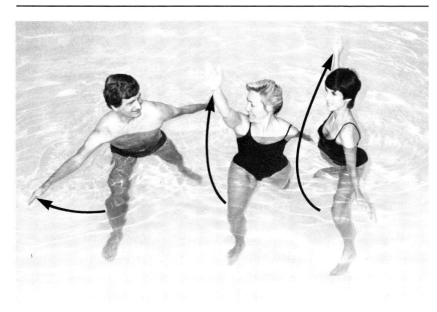

38. UP AND OVER EASY

Flex your elbows slightly as you alternately swing right and left arms forwards and backwards below the water level. Be sure each arm passes your body on the backswing to the same degree it does when it swings forwards. Repeat three or four times before you gradually raise your arms above the water level, reaching a little higher with each swing until your arms move directly overhead. Now continue the alternating motion in a full circle by moving your arms backwards, past your head until they return to your thighs. Reverse the circle. (Walk in place as you swing your arms to get even more benefit.) This exercise is felt mainly in the shoulders.

CAUTION *People with heart problems must be aware of the extra stress on the heart during this exercise. Omit it if you experience any pain or dizziness, or at your physician's recommendation.*

39. ROCK 'N ROLL

With your feet about 6 inches apart, roll forward on to your toes while you tense the muscles in your legs. Be sure to keep your head and shoulders straight and your tummy tucked in as you slowly count to six. Your arms may be spread comfortably to help maintain your balance. Now rock back on your heels until your toes are slightly raised. Count to six again, still keeping your head straight and stomach muscles tightened. Repeat. You will feel the effects of this exercise in your legs, ankles, and feet.

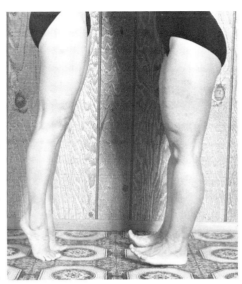

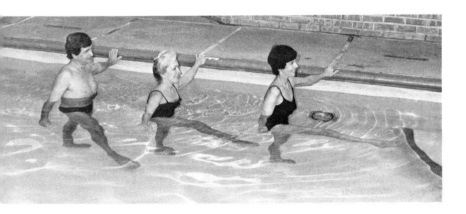

40. LEG WRITING*

With your left hand on the side for stability, right arm at your side, lift your straight right leg and write the numbers *1* to *10* by moving your leg up and down. The motion comes from your hip, so keep your knee straight. Turn round and repeat the exercise with your left leg. You may feel a stretch in your active hip and leg.

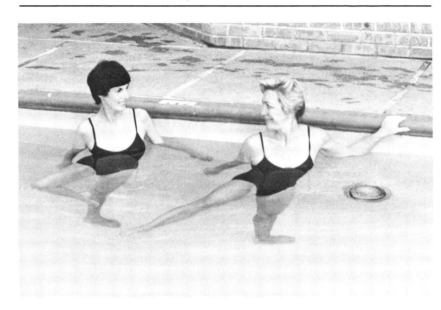

41. BENT-KNEE SIDE STRETCH

Bend and lift your right leg, knee pointing sideways as far as comfortable. Straighten your leg by gently kicking to the side. Rebend your knee before returning your foot to the pool bottom. You may brace your body against the side of the pool if you need a lot of stability, or you may rest one hand on the side if this position is more comfortable. Repeat. Do the exercise with your left leg. The hip and inside thigh of your active leg may feel a stretch.

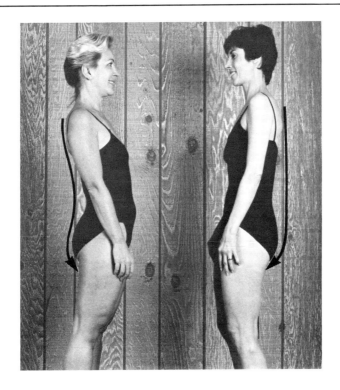

42. BACK FLATTENER*

As you stand with your feet several inches apart, knees flexed, arms at your sides, squeeze the cheeks of your buttocks together. You will notice a tendency for your pelvis to rotate forwards and upwards. Your lower back will flatten out. (It may take a little practice before the rotational motion is as pronounced as that in the photo, but don't give up.) The tighter you squeeze the flatter your back will become. Hold the position for a count of six. Relax your buttock muscles completely and repeat.

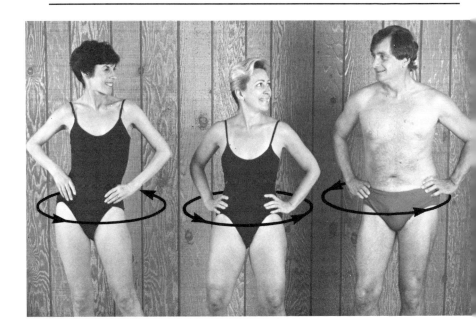

43. BELLY DANCE

Your feet are shoulder width apart, knees slightly flexed, hands on your hips. Move your hips in a wide circle, beginning to the right. Try not to move your shoulders. All the motion is underwater. Make sure that when you get to the front of the circle that the motion includes the back flattener (squeeze your buttock muscles). Do a number of repetitions before you reverse the circle. The effects may be felt in your chest, stomach, and back.

CAUTION *If you have a bad back, or if you experience any pain in your back while doing this exercise, make smaller circles or omit the exercise entirely.*

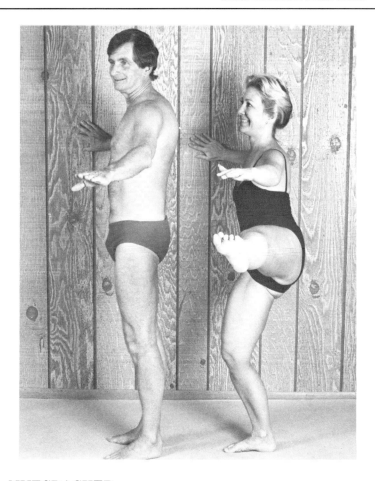

44. NUTCRACKER

Stand with your feet together, right side parallel to the edge of the pool with your right hand on the edge for stability. Your left arm may be spread to the side for further stability. Lift your left leg sideways as far as you can comfortably, and then return it to the starting position. To get added benefit from the natural resistance of the water, push your leg upwards quickly and forcefully, and then snap it back down. Repeat. Switch sides and continue the exercise. You may feel a pull in your inner thigh, hip, or knee.

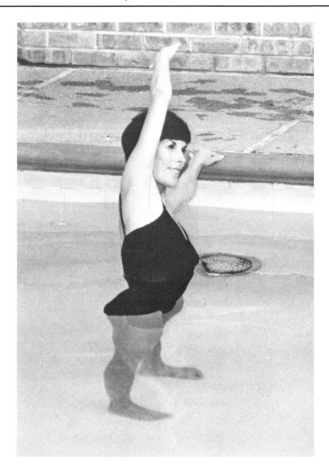

45. BALLET STRETCH

Stand with your feet comfortably apart, left side parallel to the edge of the pool. With your right arm at your side, palm up, elbow slightly flexed, lift your right arm over your head as you bend sideways to the left. Stretch as far as you can comfortably. You will feel a pull on the right side of your body. Return to the upright position, making sure that you swing your right arm all the way back down to your side. Repeat, then switch sides.

CAUTION *If you have a bad back, or if you experience any pain in your back while doing this exercise, decrease the bend or omit the exercise entirely.*

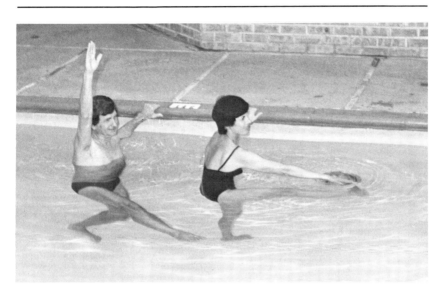

46. TOE TOUCH

Your left side is parallel to the edge of the pool as you support yourself with your left hand. Your left leg may be flexed for comfort as you lift your straight right arm over your head and swing your straight right leg forward. Bend at the waist and bring your arm down to touch your toes. Return your arm to the overhead position and your foot to the bottom. You may feel a pull in your waist, back, or thigh. Repeat, and then switch sides.

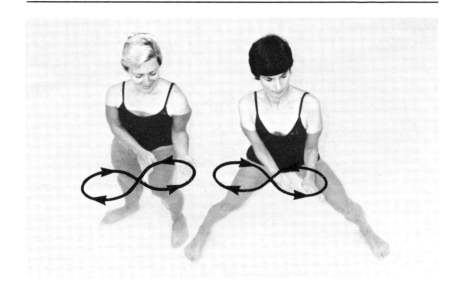

47. ORCHESTRA LEADER*

With your feet comfortably apart, flex your knees so that you
sink down until your shoulders are near the water. Keep your
back straight. Begin with your elbows touching your sides.
Pretend you are conducting a small orchestra and make a
sideways horizontal figure 8 with your palms facing each other.
Your forearms and wrists will move, but your elbows are still
touching your sides. This motion may take a little practice, but
your coordination will improve. Now reverse your figure 8. You
will feel the rotation in your wrists.

   After a while, imagine that lots more musicians join the group
and the orchestra grows very large. Continue your motion but
take your elbows away from your sides so that you use your full
arms up to the shoulder to make the figure 8s much larger. Your
hands should be well above shoulder height as they reach the
highest part of the figure. They will come through the water on
the downstroke. Reverse the motion. You may feel pressure on
your shoulders.

CAUTION *People with heart problems must be aware of the extra
stress on the heart when you lift your arms higher than your
head. You may wish to keep the figure 8s smaller, or omit the
latter part of the exercise completely.*

48. CHARLIE CHAPLIN SHRUG*

With your feet spaced comfortably apart and your back straight, sink down until your chin is near the water. Keep both arms straight against your sides. Lift your shoulders in an exaggerated shrug. Relax and repeat.

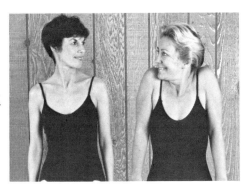

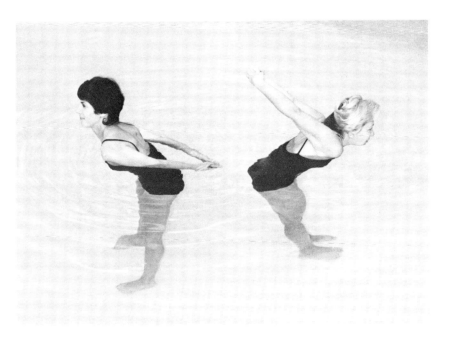

49. ORIENTAL BOW

With your feet comfortably apart, grasp your hands behind your back. Bow forwards from the waist as far as you can. Keep your head up and out of the water. Lift your arms upwards behind you, gently. Do not unclasp your hands. Return to the upright position and repeat. You may feel it in your shoulders.

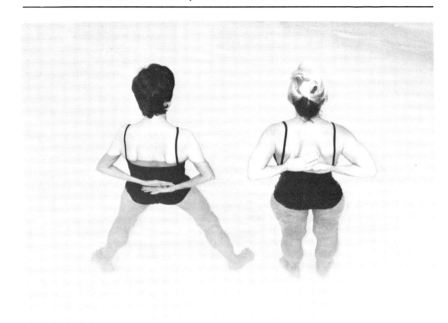

50. CLIMB THE LADDER*

Maintain your upright position, feet comfortably apart, hands behind your back. Place the back of your left hand next to, and directly above, your right in the centre of your spine. Now place your right hand just above the left. Alternate hands, climbing as high up your back as you are able. Don't forget to climb back down before you repeat the exercise. The stress here is on shoulders and upper arms.

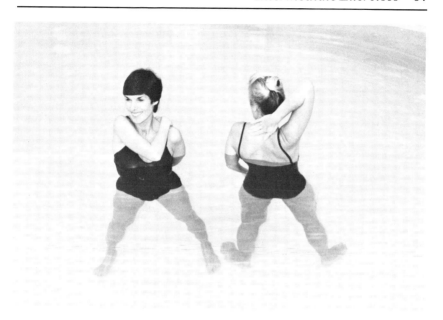

51. BACK PAT*

Place your feet comfortably apart as your right hand reaches across the front of your body and over your left shoulder. Pat gently. Return your arm to your side and then make the same motion with your left hand. Repeat.

Now your right hand reaches *behind* your head and over your right shoulder. It returns to your side when you perform the same motions with your left hand. Repeat. This exercise is generally felt in your shoulders.

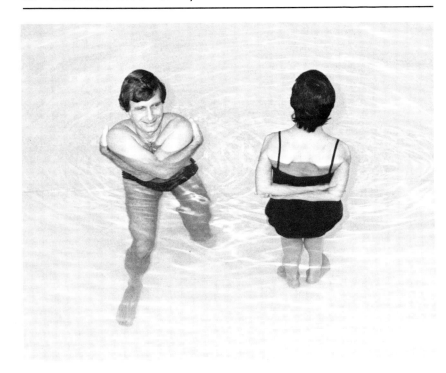

52. THE CUDDLE*

Stand comfortably. Cross your arms in front of your body until
your hands reach the opposite shoulders. Now open your arms
and move them behind your back. Grasp each elbow with the
opposite hand, or as close to the elbow as you can manage.
Repeat. You will feel the motion in your back as well as in your
shoulders and elbows.

53. COME-TO-ME*

Make sure your elbows are in the water. Keep your back straight, feet comfortably apart. Extend your arms so that they brush your thighs in front of you, palms forward, fingers straight. Gradually make a fist with your right hand while it is still in the water as you bend your right elbow to move your hand to touch your right shoulder. As you extend your right arm forward again, open your hand in the water, while bringing your left fist to your left shoulder. Continue this alternating beckoning motion. It will exercise your elbows and your fingers.

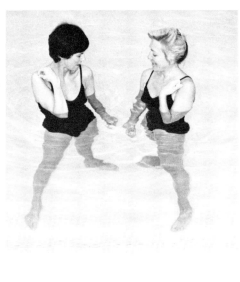

54. PRAYING HANDS*

Stand comfortably. Keep your upper arms against your sides as you bend your elbows and press your palms together. Spread your straight fingers as far apart as you can, and then bring them together again. Your hands should be *under the water*. Repeat.

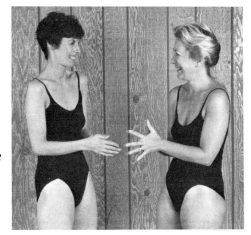

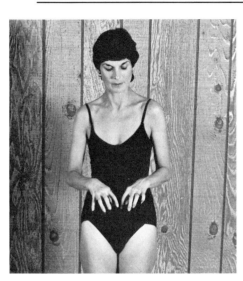

55. CAT CLAWS*

While your hands are under the water, feet comfortably apart, bend and straighten the two joints at the ends of your fingers and the end joint of your thumb, as if you were imitating a cat's clawing motion. Relax and repeat.

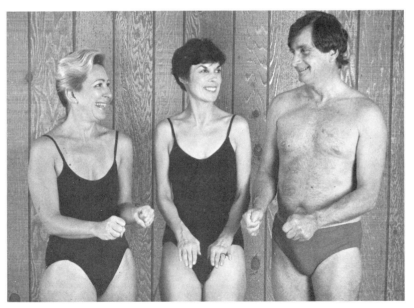

56. MAKE A FIST*

Standing comfortably with your hands underwater, open and close your fists, alternately putting your thumbs outside your fingers and then inside.

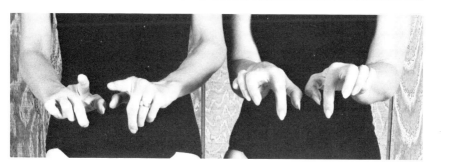

57. PIANO SOLO*

Imagine that you are seated at a piano, but continue to stand comfortably. Your thumbs strike the first notes, your index fingers lift and lower to strike the second notes, and so on until you reach your little fingers. Then work backwards towards your thumbs and repeat. Turn your palms up and continue the motion. Keep your fingers underwater.

58. SPREAD AND CLOSE*

Stand comfortably with your palms facing down, underwater. Spread your fingers apart as far as you can and then snap them back together. Keep your hands and fingers straight. Repeat.

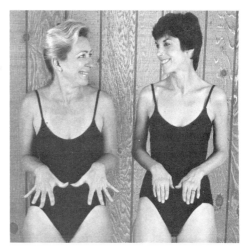

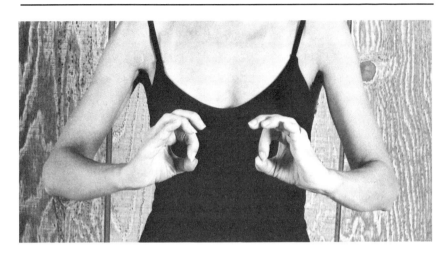

59. A-OK*

As you continue to stand comfortably, your thumb touches each rounded fingertip in turn to form a large, round letter *O*. Repeat, keeping your fingers under the water.

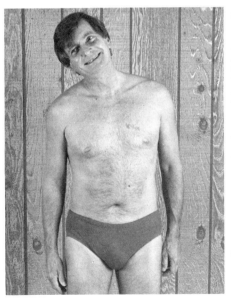

60. EAR TO SHOULDER*

Stand comfortably in the water, your arms at your sides. Be sure to keep your back straight as you drop your head to the right, as if to touch your right shoulder. Your shoulder must be relaxed. Resist the temptation to raise it. Alternate left and right sides.

CAUTION *Because your neck is a very delicate area, we strongly recommend you to check with your doctor before performing this exercise.*

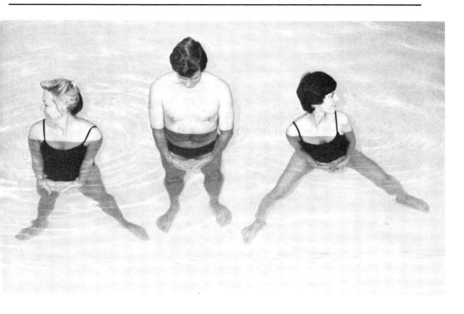

61. CHIN ROLL*

Stand comfortably, arms at your sides, fingers loosely interlaced. Bring your chin as close to your right shoulder as possible by turning your head to the right. Your chin should be parallel to the floor. Now move your chin in an arc downwards and across your chest, until it almost touches your left shoulder. Don't look up. Your chin again should be parallel to the floor. Reverse the arc, this time moving left to right. Be sure your shoulders remain down and relaxed. You will feel the motion in your neck. Repeat.

CAUTION *Because your neck is a very delicate area, we strongly recommend you to check with your doctor before performing this exercise.*

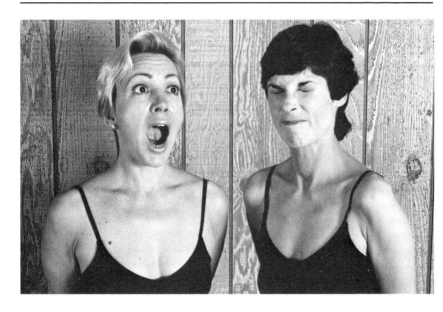

62. YAWN AND SCRUNCH*

As you continue to stand comfortably, arms at your sides, open
your mouth and eyes as wide as you possibly can in imitation of
a gigantic yawn. Now close your mouth and eyes and scrunch up
your face, tightening as many facial muscles as you can. Relax
and repeat.

Intermediate Plus

This series of exercises emphasizes total body motion and coordination. Don't give up if the exercises seem difficult at first. A little practice will do wonders.

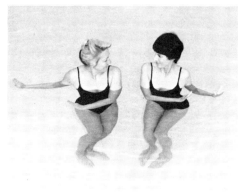

63. DISCO SKIS

Bend both elbows and shift your hands to your right side at about chest height, fingers pointing upwards. Turn both feet to the left; they should be about 4 inches apart, knees flexed. Swing your hands to the left as you pivot on your toes until they point to the right. Reverse the pivot of your hands and feet until they are back to their original positions. Keep your back straight. Repeat. Ankles, legs, hips, stomach, waist, and shoulders are all benefited.

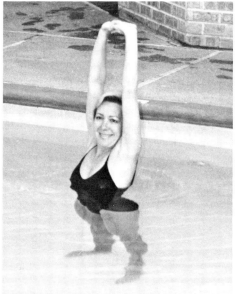

64. PALMS TO THE SKY

Stand with your feet comfortably apart, knees flexed, arms at your sides. Assume the back flattener position (exercise 42) by squeezing your buttock muscles together and rotating your pelvis and hips forward. Breathe in as you stretch your arms directly over your head, both palms upwards with one directly under the other. Hold for the count of six, exhale, and relax. You may feel a pulling in both arms and in your chest. Repeat.

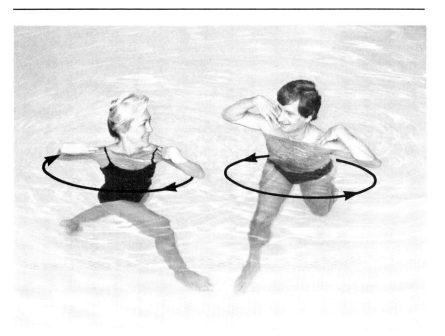

65. MOVING AGITATOR

Touch your shoulders with your fingertips, lifting your elbows up until your upper arms are parallel to the bottom, as you did in exercise 30. Flex your knees as you twist your body as far as you can to the right and then to the left. Let your head turn with your body. Your legs are placed wide apart, one foot in front of the other. After you establish a rhythm, exchange foot positions by gently jumping to shift your back foot to the front and vice versa with each twist of your body. Repeat. You may feel the movement in your shoulders, hips, and knees.

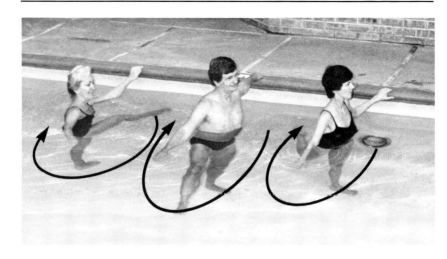

66. HALF-CIRCLE

With your left side near the wall, left hand grasping the edge, right hand extended for balance, extend your straight right leg to the front and touch the wall with your foot. Now arc that leg in a horizontal semi-circle round your body until your foot contacts the wall behind you. It's okay to bend that knee as your foot moves to the rear. Reverse the arc so that your foot travels round to the front of your body again. Repeat the whole motion. Be sure that your back is straight at all times. Turn to the other side and switch to the left leg. You may feel the motion in your back, groin, and hip.

CAUTION *If you have an artificial hip do not cross that leg in front of the other. Swing your leg only to the centre of your body.*

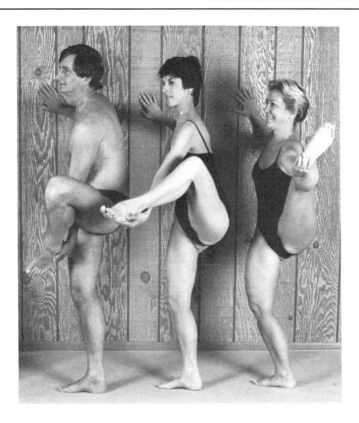

67. HEEL HOLD

With your body at a right angle to the wall, grasping the pool
edge with your right hand for support, raise your left leg and
bend your left knee. Bring your left hand down the *inside* of your
left leg and grasp your left heel. (If you can't do this exercise
while holding your heel, try holding your ankle or even your
knee.) Straighten your knee upwards and to the left side, then
bend it again and return your foot to the bottom. Repeat. Turn to
your left and switch to your right leg. You may feel a stretch in
your groin and in the back of the extended leg.

68. BALLET STRETCH WITH LEG SWING

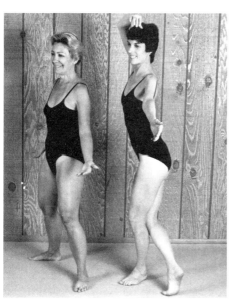

Stand with feet comfortably apart, right side parallel to the wall, arms to your sides, elbows slightly flexed, palms up. Lift your right arm over your head as you bend sideways to the left. At the same time your right foot passes behind the left, right toes touching the floor. Stretch both your right arm and leg as far to the left as is comfortable. You will feel a pull on your right side. Return to the upright position, making sure to swing your right arm all the way back down to your side. Repeat, then turn round and stretch your left arm and leg.

CAUTION *If you experience any back pain, decrease the bend or omit the exercise entirely.*

69. BODY STRETCH

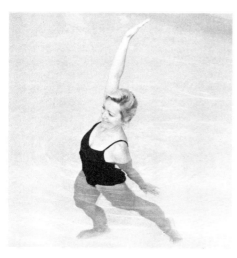

Stretch your right arm to the ceiling while you point your left foot behind you. Your left arm remains at your side, while your toe remains on the floor. Alternate your arms and legs so that your left arm stretches upwards and your right foot points to the rear. Don't rush the movements. They should be slow and deliberate. You may feel a stretch in your chest and back.

The following exercises require you to use the sides of the pool or, if you prefer, flotation devices (floats). Many people with arthritis experience pain in the small joints of their hands and fingers, so if you choose to use the edge of the pool, we urge you to drape your elbows or wrists over the edge of the pool instead of trying to grasp the edge with your fingers.

The floats used for this exercise set can be inner tubes, Styrofoam boards, or even gallon detergent containers with an inch or so of water in the bottom as ballast. If you are exceptionally unstable in the water, you may prefer to stand with your back to the side of the pool and drape your elbows and wrists over the edge. Positioning yourself in the corner of the pool makes it easier. If you feel pain in your shoulders or elbows while in this position you must stop immediately.

Remember, too, it never hurts to let the attendant know what you are up to, even though all these exercises can be done in shallow water.

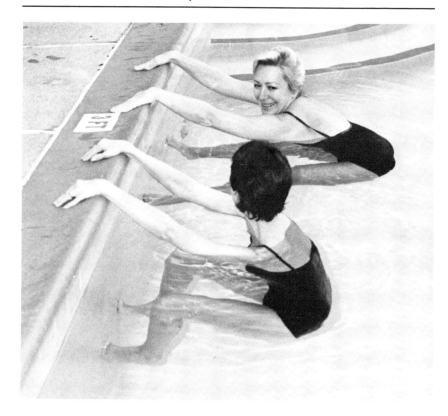

70. BABY BOUNCE

Stretch your arms forward and drape your wrists over the pool's
edge. With your legs spread comfortably, bend your knees and
put your toes on the wall a foot or two from the bottom. Let your
own level of comfort be your guide to how far up the wall you
wish to go. Do not try to keep your entire foot against the wall
while performing this exercise because it will cause too much
strain on the muscles in the backs of your legs. Bounce your
buttocks up and down by straightening and bending your knees.
Repeat. You will feel a stretch in the backs of your legs.

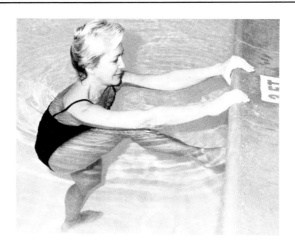

71. WALL JUMPING

Stretch your arms forward and gently grasp the pool edge. Bend your right knee and put the toes of your right foot on the wall as high as is comfortable. Your left foot stays on the floor. Bounce gently as you alternate your foot positions so that the toes of your left foot are on the wall and your right foot flat against the wall. Repeat. You may feel this exercise in your arms, waist, and the backs of your legs.

72. PUSH AND PULL

Stretch your arms forward and position your hands at the pool edge, your feet on the floor a comfortable distance apart. Let yourself move forward to the wall by bending your elbows. Then straighten them to push yourself back straight. Repeat. Your arms, wrists, and backs of your legs may feel this motion.

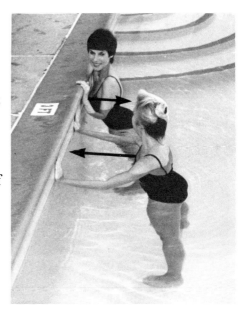

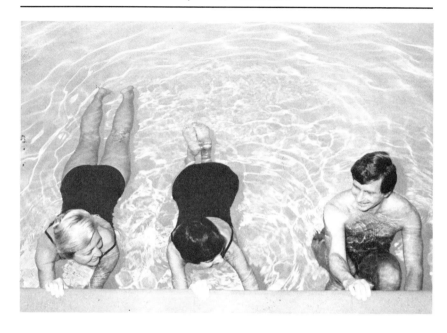

73. BODY FLOAT

Gently grasp the pool edge with your right hand and position your left hand on the wall slightly below it. Let your buttocks and extended legs float up behind you near the surface of the water. Slowly bend your knees to your chest. Your buttocks will move forward and down naturally. Finish with the toes of both feet against the wall, knees pulled as tightly to your chest as is comfortable. Repeat without letting your feet touch the bottom. Instead, push off from the wall with bent knees. Do this exercise slowly and deliberately. Don't thrust your legs backwards or forwards vigorously. You may feel a stretch in your lower back.

CAUTION *Omit this exercise if you have back pain.*

74. WALL WALK

Stretch your arms forward and gently grasp the pool edge. Walk up the wall on the balls of your feet. Your knees will bend and move higher and closer to your chest and your chin as you proceed up the wall. Go as high as you can, then walk back down. Repeat. You may feel a stretch in your lower back.

CAUTION *Omit this exercise if you have back pain.*

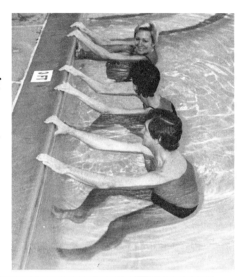

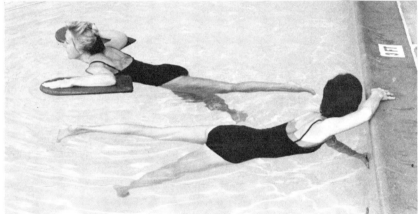

75. FRONT FLUTTER KICK

Using floats for buoyancy, or resting your hands comfortably on the side or edge of the pool if you prefer, lie on your stomach and kick your legs. Don't be concerned if you have a problem moving forwards, or even if you move backwards. Just be sure you kick from the hips rather than from the knees. It's the exercise that counts, not the distance you travel. Your shoulders, stomach, hips, thighs, knees, and the backs of your legs may feel this movement.

CAUTION *Omit this exercise if you have back pain.*

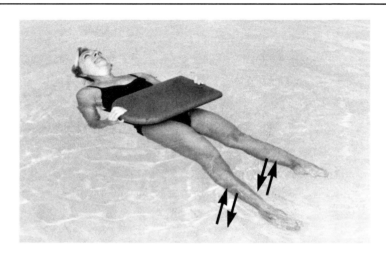

76. BACK FLUTTER KICK*

Lie on your back and hug one float to your stomach. Don't hold it behind your head. Don't try to hold the pool edge to do this exercise. Kick up and down from your hips, not your knees. Don't be concerned if you don't move forward. Good swimmers may prefer to put the float aside. You may experience tightening in your stomach, thighs, backs of your legs, hips, and knees.

77. HIP LIFT*

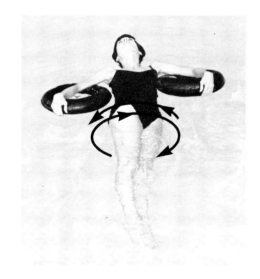

Put a float under each arm as you lie on your back, legs together and stretched forward. Twist to the right and left so that each hip rises out of the water. You may feel an effect in your waist and chest.

CAUTION *Omit this exercise if you have back pain.*

78. BICYCLE

Put a float under each arm or drape your elbows and hands over the pool edge with your back and buttocks flat against the wall. Lift both feet and imagine you are pedalling a bicycle by alternately bending and straightening each knee. Be sure to keep your upper body vertical as if you were actually sitting on a bicycle seat. Resist the urge to bend forward or to let your buttocks float forward and up. Reverse the motion by imagining that you are pedalling backwards. Your stomach, legs, and knees may feel the results of this motion.

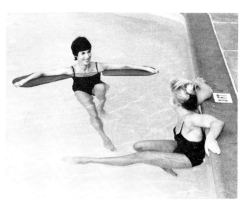

79. THE SPLITS

Put a float under each arm or drape your elbows and hands over the pool edge with your back and buttocks flat against the wall. Lift both legs and imagine that you are sitting in a chair with your legs elevated until they are parallel to the floor. Be sure your upper body is vertical. Don't lean forward and don't let your buttocks float forward and up. Point your toes up as you spread both legs as wide as you can. Then snap them together as your toes stretch forward. The water resistance you feel may act on your hips, knees, and ankles.

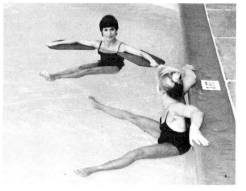

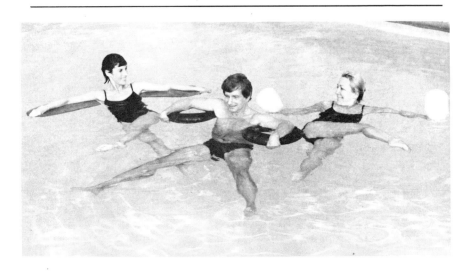

80. SCISSORS SPREAD

Put a float under each arm as you lie on your back. Keeping your legs straight, cross them, passing the left over the right as far as it will go. It's okay to lift your hip up to enable you to get the maximum leg stretch. Now shift your hips to match the angle of your shoulders and assume a sitting position with your buttocks underneath you while you spread your legs wide apart in a V position. Roll your hips forwards, and upwards if you wish, while you cross your right leg over the left as far as you can. Repeat. You may feel this exercise in your stomach, hips, and legs.

CAUTION   *If you have an artificial hip do not cross that leg over the other. Swing it only to the centre of your body. You may do the exercise as described on the side that has not had the operation.*

5
Advanced Exercises
(For Swimmers Only)

If you can do the 'Intermediate' and 'Intermediate Plus' exercises, and you are not afraid to get your face wet or to swim in deep water, you can continue with these exercises. Remember, this set is not meant for anyone who doesn't have the ability or stamina to swim at least one length (25 yards) of a standard-size swimming pool. You will need your floats for some of these exercises. If you want to spend a little money, you can pick up a set of training paddles to wear on your hands, which will strengthen weak shoulder muscles. They are sold in most sports shops.

Swimming lengths is an excellent form of exercise and any swimming stroke you choose will increase your muscle tone and give your joints a workout. You may be forced to modify a stroke that causes pain when done the way it is generally taught, but don't feel concerned if you have to sacrifice some efficiency or gracefulness in the process.

The overhand crawl (or freestyle) increases strength and endurance most rapidly, but don't neglect the sidestroke, backstroke, and front and back breaststrokes. Each offers a slightly different stretching pattern, which will enhance your total range of motion much better than just sticking to the crawl. We

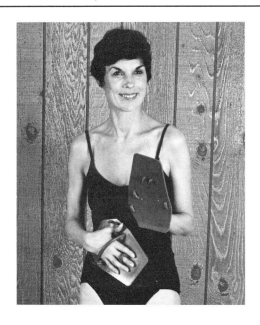

Hand paddles

don't recommend the butterfly stroke because of the unusual stress it places on the spines of even the best swimmers. If you experience any back pain when you perform the crawl it is probably because you have your head out of the water. Either swim with the accepted rhythmic breathing pattern or omit the stroke temporarily.

Before you begin this set, choose a realistic target for each exercise. Your goal can be measured by either distance or time. Increase your target gradually. Remember, steady, thoughtful movements are more important than racing tactics.

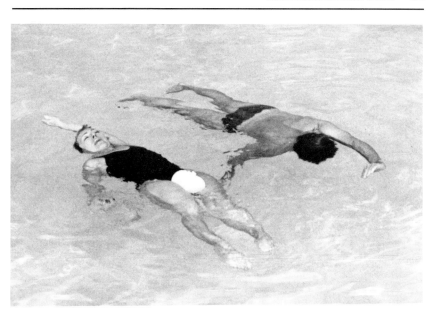

81. ARM PULL

Although swimmers' Styrofoam pull-buoys (shown in the photo), which are available in most sports shops, are ideal for performing this exercise when on your back, you can put your feet through your inner tube or simply tie two detergent containers together loosely by their handles. Grasp them between your legs comfortably. (Don't use a Styrofoam kickboard because it is too hard to hang on to.) Holding your float comfortably between your thighs (Styrofoam parts peak out above and below your thighs), swim the backstroke using just your arms and upper body. You will find that the float keeps your lower body quite high in the water. If you are a poor or average swimmer, you may choose not to use the device because it immobilizes the legs while altering your natural swimming buoyancy. Whether you use the floats or not, do not kick. All the movement comes from your arms. When you've reached the end of the pool or your target distance, turn over and do the overhand crawl without using the floats and, again, moving only your arms. Do not swim the overhand crawl with your head up.

CAUTION *Omit the overhand crawl part of this exercise if you experience back pain.*

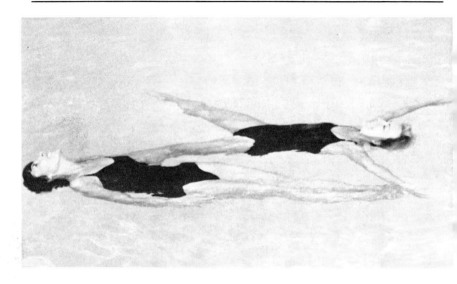

82. HORIZONTAL JUMPING JACKS

Float on your back, palms towards your body. Extend your legs.
Arc your straight arms upwards through the water until your
hands are overhead. Try to touch the backs of your hands
together if you can. At the same time, spread your straight legs.
Now pull your arms back down to your thighs while you snap
your legs together. Repeat. Shoulders, arms, hips, groin, and
legs will all feel this motion.

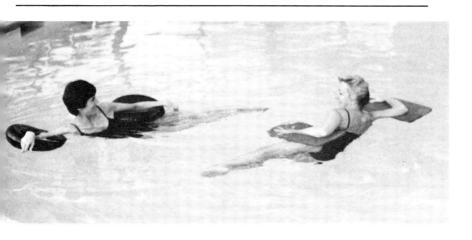

83. BICYCLE WITH A TWIST

Hold a float under each arm, making sure your buttocks are
directly underneath you, as if you were sitting in a chair. Begin
by making pedalling motions with your legs. Your upper body
faces straight ahead until you get going. Then twist your torso to
raise both legs to the left, as if you were lying on your side, and
continue to pedal. Continue for about a minute, then reverse the
direction of your legs as if you were pedalling backwards. You
will encounter some coordination difficulty the first few times
you attempt to pedal backwards, but don't get discouraged. You
still gain all the benefits of the exercise just in the attempt.

   After a minute or so, twist your body to raise your legs to the
right and pedal forwards. Continue for a minute and then
reverse-pedal. You may feel a tightening in your stomach, upper
thighs, and knees.

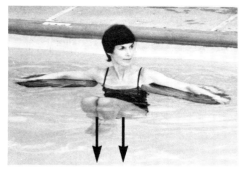

84. KNEE BENDS

The water should be at least as deep as shoulder level for this exercise. Hold a float under each arm. Your straight legs should be together beneath your body. It doesn't matter if your feet brush the bottom. Pull both knees to your chest, keeping your buttocks directly underneath you. Don't let your buttocks float forward. Now straighten your legs so that they are directly beneath you again. They should not reach forward at all. You may feel a tightening sensation in your stomach or a stretch in your lower back.

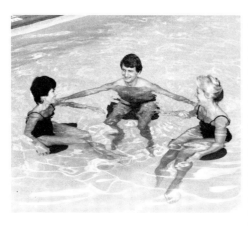

85. FREE RIDE

Balance yourself while sitting on your board or tube. (Detergent containers won't work for this exercise.) Cup your hands and pull yourself forward by reaching comfortably in front of you and pulling the water back as you circle your arms to the side as if doing a breaststroke. Try to travel the length of the pool. Now reverse the motion so that you move backwards for a length. Your shoulders, arms, and stomach will feel this motion.

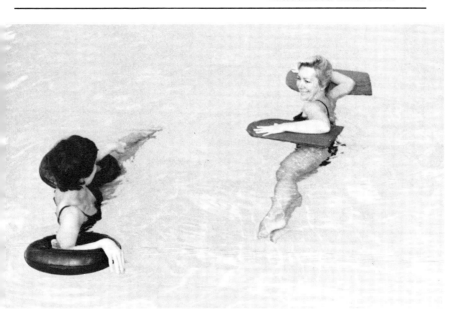

86. ADVANCED TICK-TOCK SWING

Hold a float under each arm as you balance yourself vertically, legs together beneath you. Then swing both legs from side to side without letting your buttocks or legs float forwards. Move your legs only as high as you can without pain. You'll feel a gentle pull along each side of your body as your legs swing in the opposite direction. Repeat.

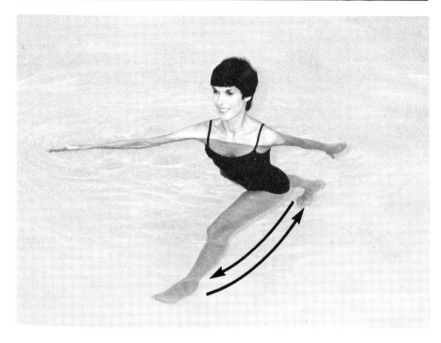

87. GIANT STEPS

Swing your legs back and forth from the hip as if you were
taking giant strides along the bottom of the pool, but stay in the
same place. You can do this in shoulder-deep water by gently
jumping on the spot as shown in the photo. You can also do this
in deep water by holding a float under each arm and swinging
your legs back and forth freely. Either way, you may feel motion
in your hips and legs.

6
Isometrics

Because isometrics work muscle against muscle or immobile object, these exercises are helpful when you are having a flare-up or your painful, inflamed joints can't tolerate the more active exercises we have shown you. When performed consistently they prevent muscle deterioration without relying on painful joint movements. Isometric exercises can be done anytime, anywhere, usually in either a standing or sitting position, and they don't require special equipment or a human helper. They don't even need to be done in the bath, although we recommend that you include them in your at-home regime.

But as valuable as isometric exercises are, they do have one big drawback. If you stop doing them without resuming other more active exercises, any strength you have managed to build will be lost in just about the same length of time that you spent developing it. The beneficial effects of the exercises we have described up to this point, known as isotonics *because they involve active motion of muscles and joints, do not disappear nearly as rapidly. Therefore, you must make the time to go through your isometric exercises several times each day, and more after you have built up some stamina. Do as many repetitions as you can.*

CAUTION *If you have high blood pressure or heart trouble, consult a physician before doing isometrics, since the exercises can temporarily inhibit circulation.*

NOTE *Exercises that can be done in a bath are marked with asterisks.*

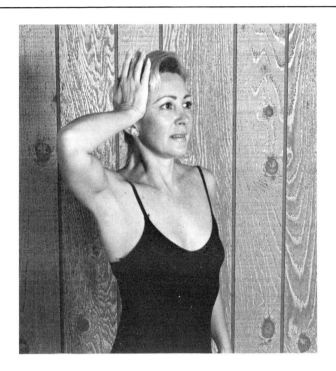

88. HEAD/HAND PRESS*

Press your right palm against the right side of your head, with
your elbow pointing sideways. Push your head towards your
hand as your hand pushes towards your head. Take a breath,
count to six slowly, exhale, and relax. Repeat. Do the same with
your left hand. Repeat. You will feel a tensing in the sides of
your neck and in your arm muscles as you press against your
head.

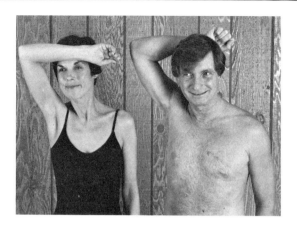

89. HEAD/FOREARM PRESS*

Lift and press your right forearm against your forehead as your head pushes your forearm with the same force. Inhale, count to six, exhale, and relax. Repeat. Put your forearm on the back of your head and push both your head and forearm with the same force. Repeat. Now perform the same exercise with your left forearm. In addition to the pressure on your head, you will feel contractions in the back and front of your neck and in your arm muscles.

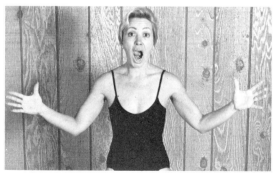

90. SILENT SHOUT*

Open your mouth as wide as you can while you inhale. Hold the position and 'shout' silently for the count of six. Exhale and relax. Repeat. You will feel tension in the joints of your jaw under your ears and in the front of your neck.

91. LAZY MAN'S PRESS*

Gently interlace your fingers behind your neck. Inhale and count to six slowly as you push your neck backwards against your hands and your hands pull forwards against your neck. Keep your elbows pointed sideways. Exhale, relax the tension, and repeat. You will feel pressure on the back of your neck and tension in your neck and arm muscles.

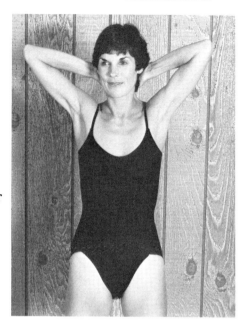

92. MILITARY SHOULDERS*

Inhale and count to six as you tighten your chest muscles while you tense your shoulders and pull them slightly backwards. Exhale and relax by bringing your shoulders to their normal position. Make sure you do not raise your shoulders during any part of this exercise and that your neck and back are straight. Repeat. You will feel tension in your chest, shoulders, and mid-back.

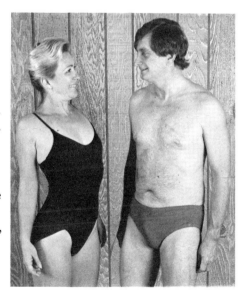

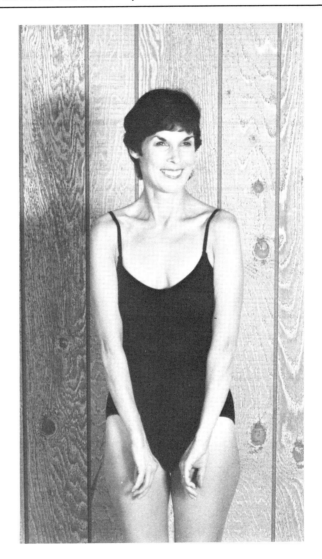

93. SHOULDER PINCH*

Inhale as you push your shoulders forward. Hold for the count of six, exhale, and relax by bringing your shoulders to their normal position. Don't raise your shoulders during this exercise and be sure that your neck and back are straight. Repeat. You will feel tension in your shoulders, mid-back area, and rib cage.

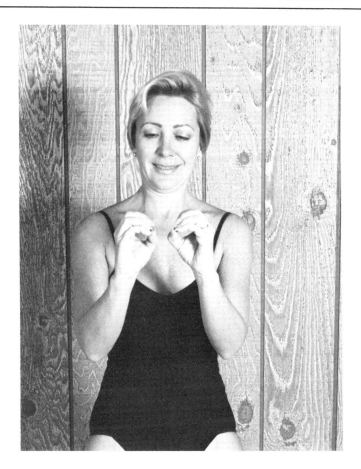

94. ROUNDED FINGERS*

Both hands work together as you press the pad of each index finger to its thumb, keeping the joints rounded. Imagine that your hands are circled round a pill bottle. Inhale, count to six, exhale, and relax. Continue by pressing each finger to its thumb in turn. Repeat. You will feel contractions in your thumbs as well as each finger and a slight tension in your wrists and forearms.

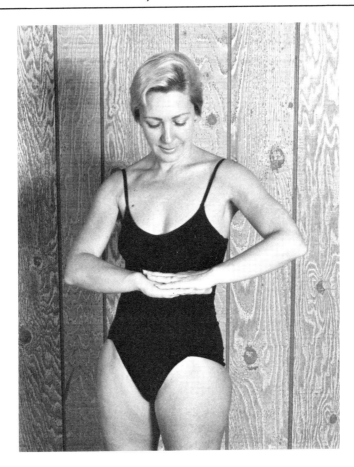

95. HAND OVER HAND*

Place your left palm over the top of your right hand at about waist level. Your hands should be comfortably away from your body. Inhale and push down with your left hand while pushing up with your right. Count to six, exhale, and relax. Reverse your hands so that the right palm is on top and repeat. You will feel tension from your hands all the way up to your shoulders and down your spine.

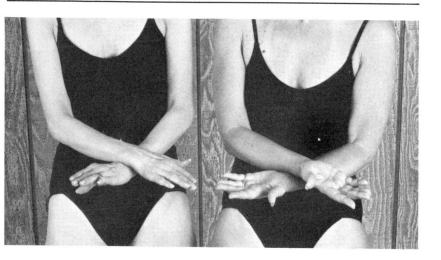

96. WRIST CROSS*

Cross your wrists and press them against each other, palms down, at waist level. Your hands should be comfortably away from your body. Inhale as you press your wrists together, count to six, exhale, and relax. Reverse crossed-wrist position and repeat. Turn your palms upwards and repeat the whole exercise. You will feel tension from your wrists to your shoulders.

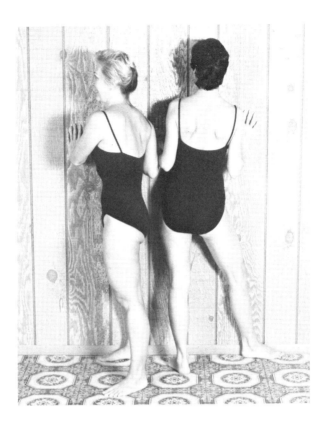

97. PUSH THE WALL

Press both hands against the wall for balance as you stand facing it. Then, turning to the left, press the outside edge of your right foot against the wall. Inhale, count to six, exhale, and relax. Again facing the wall, place the inside of your right foot against the wall and press. (You may have to shift your weight slightly.) Use your hands, elbows bent, to brace yourself against the wall. You may get added benefit by deliberately applying pressure to the wall with your hands simultaneously. Repeat. Then do the exercise with your left foot. You will feel tension in the muscles of your foot and the outside of your leg when the outside of your foot is pressed to the wall. The tension will be felt up the inside of your leg when the inside of your foot is against the wall. You will also feel tension from your wrists up your arms to your shoulders and down your mid-back.

CAUTION *Omit the deliberate pressing of your hands against the wall if you experience pain in your wrists.*

7
Exercises to Do at Home

Exercising at home is a good way to supplement your total programme. The exercises we describe can help you loosen up and start the day, relax away your tensions at the end of the day, and prepare for any special event by relieving stress and giving you a sense of well-being.

Sometimes it is inconvenient to visit the pool, and sometimes, during a flare-up, you just don't feel up to the trip. Your physician may even advise you to omit your visits to the water for a while. Yet you can maintain your level of fitness at home in your own bath. We suggest that you incorporate all the isometric exercises in chapter 6 into your at-home regimen, too, if your doctor approves.

Any exercise that we have marked with an asterisk can be done at home in a very full bath so that the muscles and joints you are exercising can be submerged as much as possible. We suggest that you do the exercises in a sitting position unless you are uncomfortable and prefer to lie down in the bath with the water level slightly decreased. If your legs are very long, you may be forced to bend your knees slightly, but this will not affect the beneficial effects of the bath exercises to any significant degree.

Be sure to do your exercises before you actually use the soap so *that you don't slide on a slippery surface. A non-skid mat or the installation of safety-strip tape is recommended. Then, too, it's good to have someone else at home,* within calling distance, *while you are exercising. In addition you should think seriously about installing a safety handrail above the bath. It will stabilize your balance while you get in and out and give you something to hang on to while you are exercising, if you need it. Don't rely on soap-dish handles. In most cases they are not secure enough to hold your weight. Be careful not to stub your toes on taps, handles, and so forth.*

Some people find a washbasin or sink, or even a bucket or two, useful for their at-home exercises. Time spent washing dishes or hand-washing can be stretched to include all the finger, thumb, hand, and wrist exercises we have already outlined, and you can even do some of the forearm and a couple of the elbow exercises. Toes, feet, and ankles can be exercised in two buckets of warm water on the bathroom or kitchen floor. Be sure there are no electric stoves or bars that could fall into the bath from the wall.

Please refer to the chart on pages 115–25, which details all the exercises in earlier chapters that can also be done at home in the bath.

NOTE *Exercises that can be done in a bath are marked with asterisks.*

98. CURLY TOES*

Curl your toes, then
relax the tension.
Repeat.

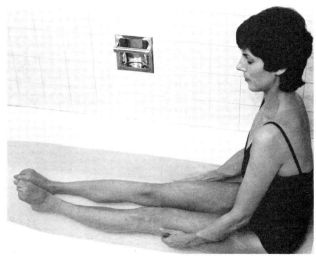

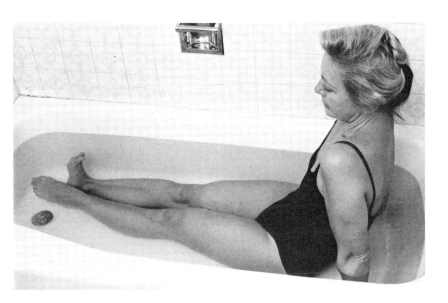

99. FOOT PEDALS*

Roll one foot towards your face while you point the other down
as far as you can. Repeat. Reverse feet and perform the exercises
again. You will feel tension in your ankles as well as in your
toes.

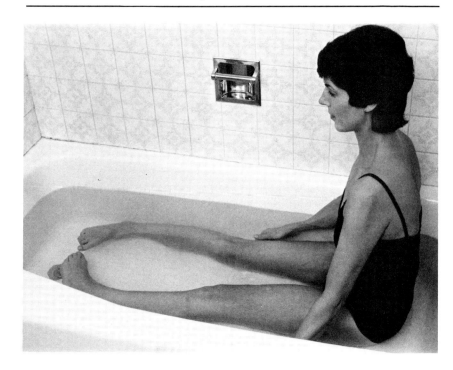

100. ANKLE CIRCLES*

Lift both feet very slightly off the bottom of the bath and circle
them inwards (towards each other) from the ankle. Repeat.
Reverse the direction. You will feel the movement in your
ankles and the backs of your legs.

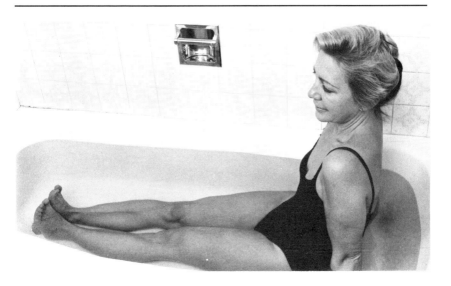

101. FOOT COUNTING*

With both your feet raised slightly off the bottom, stretch your toes straight upwards. Now trace the numeral *1* by lowering your toes as far as you can. The motion comes from the ankles, not the knees. Relax. Trace the numerals *2, 3,* etcetera, to *10* in the same manner. It is not necessary to press your knees together tightly. You will feel this exercise in your ankles and the backs of your legs.

102. ANKLE FIGURE 8*

With both your feet slightly off the bottom, point your toes to the left and trace the numeral *8* several times by circling your toes first to the right and then back to the left again. Repeat and reverse the direction.

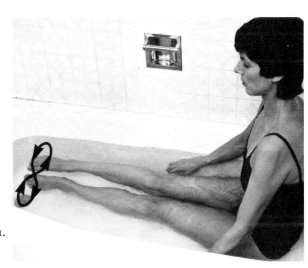

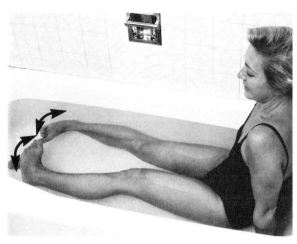

103. ARC YOUR TOES*

Spread your legs and point the toes of each foot towards the other. Now swing them away from each other as far as you can. Try to make a 180° arc. Swing them back to the original point. Repeat. You will feel rotation in your ankles.

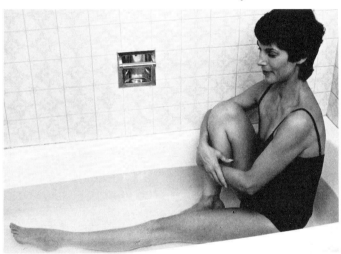

104. KNEE CUDDLE*

Be sure to keep your back straight and your head up throughout this exercise. Bend your right leg, grasp your knee and pull it to your chest. Alternate left and right knees. Your stomach and back may feel this motion.

CAUTION *People with artificial hips or knees should not pull their knees to their chests. Instead bend the knee only as much as you can comfortably without using your hands.*

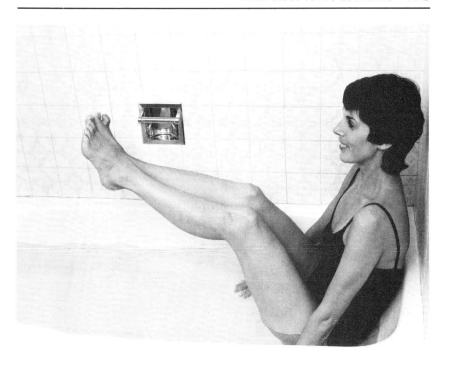

105. PERPENDICULAR LEGS*

Begin with your legs straight out in front of you, ankles
touching at all times. Bend your knees towards your chest as
you raise your feet upwards as high as you can without pain. Try
to hold for a second or two if possible. Return your legs to the
bottom as you straighten your knees. Relax. Repeat. If you
choose a sitting position for this exercise it is okay to lean back
as you raise your feet. You will feel a strong contraction in your
stomach muscles.

CAUTION *Omit this exercise if you are having back pain.*

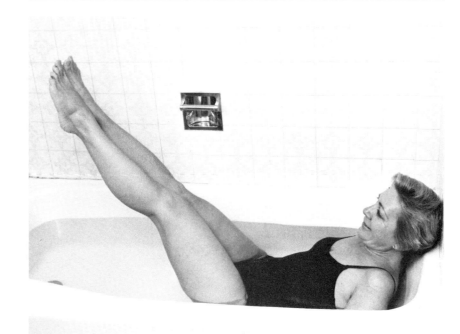

106. SKY LIFT*

With your ankles together, lift both straight legs directly upwards as far as you can without pain. Try to hold the position for a second or two before you lower them back down to the bottom of the bath. Repeat. You may cushion your spine by putting a small folded hand towel or cloth under your lower back at the hollow of your spine if you find it more comfortable, since, because of the effort required of your stomach muscles, you will probably not be able to perform this exercise in a sitting position.

CAUTION   *Omit this exercise if you are having back pain.*

EXERCISE REVIEW CHART

Use this chart as an aid for your total exercise programme. Refer to your own specific painful body areas so that you can do more repetitions of those exercises that focus on exactly where it hurts. However, we recommend that you follow a balanced exercise regimen rather than exercising *only* painful muscles and joints. This way you can reach the optimum physical fitness level for your age and physical condition.

We have listed the exercises in the order in which they appear in this book. Major joints and muscle groups are listed alphabetically. A solid circle is used to indicate appropriate exercises for specific areas.

If you feel pain in a part of your body that is not specifically mentioned in one of the columns, simply choose exercises designed for the two closest parts. For example, pain in your upper arm around the biceps will be helped by shoulder and elbow exercises. Pain in the calf should respond to movements directed towards the ankles and knees and even some for the hips.

An open circle is used when a specific muscle group or joint is not directly affected by the specific movements of the exercise but receives an important indirect benefit. As an example, many of the exercises listed in the column headed 'Back' are indicated by open circles to let you know that your back will be benefited when you exercise other muscles, such as your stomach muscles.

Don't be concerned if you are unable to do the exercises exactly as they are pictured. Do the best you can to come close to the photographs and you will still enjoy tremendous benefits.

Exercise number	Exercise name	Ankle	Back	Elbow	Fingers & hand	Groin	Head & face	Hi
1.	STICKY STRUT	●						●
2.	STRAIGHT-LEG MARCH							●
3.	BENT-LEG MARCH							●
4.	SEMI-CIRCLE STRUT					●		●
5.	SIDE-STEP SHUFFLE					●		●
6.	BACKWARDS WALK	●	○					●
7.	WAVE AT THE FISHES	●			●			
8.	ANKLE CIRCLES	●						
9.	CAN-CAN							
10.	KNEE ROCK	○						
11.	STRAIGHT-LEG SWING/FRONT TO BACK							●
12.	LEG ARC		○					●
13.	LEG CIRCLES		○			○		●
14.	MONEY TREE			●	●			
15.	CURLY FINGERS AND TOES				●			
16.	WEIGHTED THUMBS			●				
17.	ELBOW BEND			●	●			
18.	ROCKING THE BABY			●	●			
19.	VICTORY	●		●				
20.	SHOULDER ROLL				●			
21.	SIDE GLANCE							
22.	YES, YES							
23.	PICTURE FRAME			●	●			
24.	CHARLESTON	●		●				●

Knee	Neck	Shoulders	Stomach	Toes & feet	Chest & waist	Wrist	General fitness/ aerobic	Bath
●				●				
		●	○		●		●	
●		●	○				●	
			○				●	
		●	○				●	
		●		●			●	
						●		●
								●
●								
●								
			○					
			○					
	●	●		●	●			
				●				●
						○		●
						●		●
		●			●			●
●		●		●	●		●	
		●						
	●							●
	●							●
		●			○			●
●		●	○	●		●	●	

Exercise number	Exercise name	Ankle	Back	Elbow	Fingers & hand	Groin	Head & face	Hip
25.	PUSH, LIFT, BEND, AND STRETCH			●	●			
26.	KNEE-UP		●		●			
27.	KNEE SQUATS	○						●
28.	TICK-TOCK SWING					○		●
29.	WAIST TWIST		●					
30.	AGITATOR	●	●					
31.	SUPER STRETCH		●					●
32.	TAKE A BOW		●					
33.	MAE WEST							
34.	SIDE ARM LIFT			○	○			
35.	ELBOW KISS		○	●				
36.	FENCING	●		●				●
37.	KICK WALK	●						●
38.	UP AND OVER EASY	●		○				●
39.	ROCK 'N ROLL	●						
40.	LEG WRITING							●
41.	BENT-KNEE SIDE STRETCH					●		●
42.	BACK FLATTENER		●					●
43.	BELLY DANCE		●					●
44.	NUTCRACKER					○		●
45.	BALLET STRETCH		●					●
46.	TOE TOUCH	○			●			●
47.	ORCHESTRA LEADER			●	●			
48.	CHARLIE CHAPLIN SHRUG							
49.	ORIENTAL BOW		○		●			
50.	CLIMB THE LADDER			●				
51.	BACK PAT			●	●			

Knee	Neck	Shoulders	Stomach	Toes & feet	Chest & waist	Wrist	General fitness/aerobic	Bath
		●	○		○	●	●	
●		●	○		●			●
●								
				●	●			
					●			
		●		●	●			
		●	●		●			
		●						●
		●						
		●				●		
●	●	●		●			●	
●		●	○		●		●	
●		●			○		●	
			●	●				
								●
●								
●			○		●			●
			●		●			
○								
		●			●			
		●	○		●			
		●				●		●
		●						●
		●	○		●			
		●						●
		●				●		●

Exercise number	Exercise name	Ankle	Back	Elbow	Fingers & hand	Groin	Head & face	Hi
52.	THE CUDDLE		○	●	●			
53.	COME-TO-ME			●	●			
54.	PRAYING HANDS			●	●			
55.	CAT CLAWS				●			
56.	MAKE A FIST				●			
57.	PIANO SOLO				●			
58.	SPREAD AND CLOSE				●			
59.	A-OK				●			
60.	EAR TO SHOULDER							
61.	CHIN ROLL							
62.	YAWN AND SCRUNCH						●	
63.	DISCO SKIS	●	○		○			●
64.	PALMS TO THE SKY		○	○	●			
65.	MOVING AGITATOR	●	●	○	○			●
66.	HALF-CIRCLE	○	○			●		●
67.	HEEL HOLD		○	●	●	○		●
68.	BALLET STRETCH WITH LEG SWING	●	●	●				●
69.	BODY STRETCH	●	●					●
70.	BABY BOUNCE		○					●
71.	WALL JUMPING	●	○					●
72.	PUSH AND PULL			●				
73.	BODY FLOAT		●	●				●
74.	WALL WALK	●	○	●				●
75.	FRONT FLUTTER KICK	●	○			●		●
76.	BACK FLUTTER KICK	●	○			●		●
77.	HIP LIFT		●					

Knee	Neck	Shoulders	Stomach	Toes & feet	Chest & waist	Wrist	General fitness/ aerobic	Bath
		●				●		●
								●
					●			●
								●
								●
								●
								●
	●							●
								●
●		●	●	●	●			
		●			○	●		
●		○	○	●	●		●	
●			○		○			
●		●	○					
		●	○	●	●			
		●	○	●	●			
●	○				●			
●		●		●	●			
		●		●		○		
●		●	●	●		●		
●		●	○	●				
●		●	○				●	
●			○				●	●
			○		●			●

Exercise number	Exercise name	Ankle	Back	Elbow	Fingers & hand	Groin	Head & face	Hi
78.	BICYCLE	●	○					●
79.	THE SPLITS	○	○			●		●
80.	SCISSORS SPREAD		○			●		●
81.	ARM PULL		○	●	●			
82.	HORIZONTAL JUMPING JACKS				●	●		
83.	BICYCLE WITH A TWIST	●	○					●
84.	KNEE BENDS		●					●
85.	FREE RIDE			●	●			
86.	ADVANCED TICK-TOCK SWING		●					
87.	GIANT STEPS							●
88.	HEAD/HAND PRESS			○			●	
89.	HEAD/FOREARM PRESS			○				
90.	SILENT SHOUT						●	
91.	LAZY MAN'S PRESS			○	●		●	
92.	MILITARY SHOULDERS		●					
93.	SHOULDER PINCH		●					
94.	ROUNDED FINGERS			○	●			
95.	HAND OVER HAND			○	●			
96.	WRIST CROSS			○				
97.	PUSH THE WALL	●	○	○	●	●		●
98.	CURLY TOES	●						
99.	FOOT PEDALS	●						
100.	ANKLE CIRCLES	●						
101.	FOOT COUNTING	●						

Knee	Neck	Shoulders	Stomach	Toes & feet	Chest & waist	Wrist	General fitness/ aerobic	Bath
●			○				●	
○			○	●				
			○		●			
	●	●			●	●	●	
		●					●	
●			●		●		●	
●			●					
		●	○			●	●	
			○		●			
				○				
	●	○				●		●
	●	○						●
	●							●
	●	○						●
		●			●			●
		●			●			●
						○		●
		○			●	○		●
		○				●		●
●		●		●		●		
				●				●
				○				●
○								●
				●				●

Exercise number	Exercise name	Ankle	Back	Elbow	Fingers & hand	Groin	Head & face	Hip
102.	ANKLE FIGURE 8	●						
103.	ARC YOUR TOES	●						●
104.	KNEE CUDDLE		○	●	●			●
105.	PERPENDICULAR LEGS		○					●
106.	SKY LIFT		○					●

Knee	Neck	Shoulders	Stomach	Toes & feet	Chest & waist	Wrist	General fitness/ aerobic	Bath
				●				●
○								●
●		●	○					●
●			●					●
			●					●

INDEX